# BestMasters

Mit „BestMasters" zeichnet Springer die besten Masterarbeiten aus, die an renommierten Hochschulen in Deutschland, Österreich und der Schweiz entstanden sind. Die mit Höchstnote ausgezeichneten Arbeiten wurden durch Gutachter zur Veröffentlichung empfohlen und behandeln aktuelle Themen aus unterschiedlichen Fachgebieten der Naturwissenschaften, Psychologie, Technik und Wirtschaftswissenschaften. Die Reihe wendet sich an Praktiker und Wissenschaftler gleichermaßen und soll insbesondere auch Nachwuchswissenschaftlern Orientierung geben.

Springer awards "BestMasters" to the best master's theses which have been completed at renowned Universities in Germany, Austria, and Switzerland. The studies received highest marks and were recommended for publication by supervisors. They address current issues from various fields of research in natural sciences, psychology, technology, and economics. The series addresses practitioners as well as scientists and, in particular, offers guidance for early stage researchers.

Hannah Eger

# Feminist Global Health Policy

Addressing Health Inequalities through an Intersectional Perspective

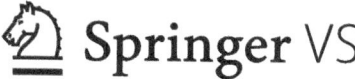 Springer VS

Hannah Eger
Faculty of Sociology, Bielefeld
University
School of Public Health, Bielefeld
University
Berlin, Germany

This thesis was approved by the School of Public Health and Faculty of Sociology at Bielefeld University to obtain the academic degrees of Master of Science in Public Health and Master of Arts in Political Science.

ISSN 2625-3577                    ISSN 2625-3615   (electronic)
BestMasters
ISBN 978-3-658-43496-0          ISBN 978-3-658-43497-7   (eBook)
https://doi.org/10.1007/978-3-658-43497-7

This Springer VS imprint is published by the registered company Springer Fachmedien Wiesbaden GmbH, part of Springer Nature.
The registered company address is: Abraham-Lincoln-Str. 46, 65189 Wiesbaden, Germany

Paper in this product is recyclable.

# Acknowledgement

*It is in collectivities that we find reservoirs of hope and optimism.*
*(Angela Y. Davis, 2016, p. 49)*

I want to express my profound gratitude to Awa Naghipour, Charisse Jordan, Deborah Leticia Akumu, Emma Rhule, Jonathan Cohen, Marie Meudec, Oriana López Uribe, Salma El-Gamal, Sandhya Kanaka Yatirajula, Shehnaz Munshi, and Shubha Chacko. This thesis would not have been possible without their participation in the focus groups that ultimately informed the findings. I would like to further thank everyone who supported me in the process of researching and writing this thesis.

# Abstract

**Background:** Health inequalities, primarily driven by the structural determinants of health, are a major concern towards the global goal of health for all. The political level is essential for health equality since it highly influences these determinants, including gender, race, and class. Structurally embedded power hierarchies cause intersecting positions of privilege and oppression, resulting in health inequalities and adverse health outcomes. A feminist global health policy addresses the unequal distribution of power and focuses on the marginalised to dismantle power hierarchies. Prioritising an intersectional, holistic, human rights-based approach intends to mitigate health inequalities.

**Research objective:** The objective of this research is to identify what a feminist global health policy encompasses and how it can be implemented in practice, by elaborating a framework for a feminist global health policy.

**Methodology:** Three online focus groups were conducted via Zoom in August and September 2022. Through purposive sampling, participants affiliated to either the global-academic or local-activist level were included, envisaging global representation. A participatory approach was employed consistent with feminist research principles. Subjectivity and lived experience were acknowledged in alignment with a postmodern epistemology. Based on qualitative content analysis by Kuckartz, ten main codes and 25 subcodes were identified.

**Results:** The framework for a feminist global health policy is centred on the concept of intersectionality and considerations of power and knowledge. It provides a nexus between the global and the local level, by entailing universal principles as well as recommendations and sensitivity for context-specific adaptations. Community and policymakers are identified as the main actors, with the latter being accountable. The adoption of this framework is anticipated to contribute to addressing current challenges in global health and progress towards health equality and reproductive justice.

**Conclusion:** A feminist global health policy requires a paradigm shift. Albeit being an intricate process, its implementation is not impossible. Continuous work towards the vision of health equality is imperative to eventually translate it into practice.

# Contents

# Abbreviations

| | |
|---|---|
| AAAQ | Availability, accessibility, acceptability, and quality |
| AU | African Union |
| BIPoC | Black, Indigenous, and People of Colour |
| CEDAW | Convention on the Elimination of All Forms of Discrimination against Women |
| CFFP | Centre for Feminist Foreign Policy |
| EU | European Union |
| FGHP | Feminist global health policy |
| GBV | Gender-based violence |
| HICs | High-income countries |
| LICs | Low-income countries |
| LIMCs | Low-and-middle-income countries |
| SDG | Sustainable Development Goal |
| SDOH | Social determinants of health |
| SRHR | Sexual and reproductive health and rights |
| STI | Sexually-transmitted infection |
| UN | United Nations |
| WHO | World Health Organization |

# List of Figures

# List of Tables

# Introduction

> *Of all the forms of inequality, injustice in health is the most shocking and the most inhuman because it often results in physical death.*

(Martin Luther King, 1966)

> *There is no thing as a single-issue struggle because we do not live single-issue lives.*

(Audre Lorde, 1984, p. 138)

The harmful consequences of health inequalities are far from new (e.g. White-head & Burström, 2021; Yao et al., 2019). In a speech in 1966, the Black[1] human rights activist Martin Luther King Jr. emphasised their life-threatening risks. By referring to "injustice", King (1966) endorsed that these inequalities are avoidable since they stem from human-made inequities. Health inequities are structurally embedded. They originate from power asymmetries determined by the socioeconomic-political context (Marmot & Allen, 2014; Solar & Irwin, 2010). As the Black feminist Audre Lorde (1984) alluded to, the world is complex. Accordingly, multiple power regimes exist and are interconnected, causing intersecting forms of privileges and oppression (Crenshaw, 1989; Hill Collins,

---

[1] In this thesis, Black is capitalised when referring to Black people. Black does not refer to a colour, but to a shared identity. Furthermore, it serves as a self-designation and form of empowerment against the backdrop of the brutal history of oppression. In this respect, white is written in lowercase to avoid reproduction of white supremacy. This approach is consistent with a postmodern understanding that emphasises language (e.g. Eggers et al., 2005; Mohamed, 2022).

H. Eger, *Feminist Global Health Policy*, BestMasters, https://doi.org/10.1007/978-3-658-43497-7_1

2019). For instance, discrimination on the basis of gender, race, and class generates inequalities with corresponding implications for health (Hill Collins, 2019). An intersectional understanding highlights the multidimensionality of intertwined power regimes, i.e. a white poor women is differently affected than a Black transgender man (Carastathis, 2014; Davis, 1981). Moreover, the world is characterised by globalisation, enhancing its complexity. Power hierarchies and resulting adverse health outcomes persist and are reproduced globally (Chancel et al., 2021; Hill Collins, 2000).

However, the preventability of structural inequalities due to their social constructiveness implies that they can be challenged and changed (Solar & Irwin, 2010). In accordance with Lorde (1984) this requires an intersectional approach. The political level as well as "the conditions in which people are born, grow, work, live, and age" (WHO, 2022, para. 1), referred to as the social determinants of health (SDOH), must be acknowledged. The impact of living conditions and the environment on health has been recognised by Indigenous knowledge long before the SDOH were designated (Greenwood & Lindsay, 2019; Nettleton et al., 2007).

A feminist global health policy (FGHP) intends to provide an alternative with the objective to improve health and well-being for all. By incorporating a holistic, intersectional approach, power hierarchies are to be dismantled and structural inequalities eliminated (CFFP, 2021; Davies et al., 2019). With reference to King (1966), addressing health inequities to achieve equality is of major importance for the survival of individuals as well as society.

Feminist approaches to global health policy demand transformation and new ways of thinking (CFFP, 2021). In this regard, this thesis serves to elaborate a framework for a FGHP. The intention is to identify what such an approach encompasses and how it can be meaningfully incorporated, with respect to global principles as well as context-specific circumstances. Due to its interdisciplinary nature, this topic is of considerable relevance to the disciplines of public health as well as political science.

To introduce the topic and relevant literature, extensive information about health inequalities and the concept of intersectionality are presented, with particular emphasis on the structural determinants gender, race, and class (Chapter 2). For a comprehensive understanding, examples of the implications for health and well-being are provided. Previous and current political endeavours towards equality at multilateral level are highlighted in Chapter 3, followed by an introduction to a feminist approach to global health policy. Subsequently, the research interest and question derived from the reviewed literature is depicted (Chapter 4). The methodology of the present research is outlined in Chapter 5, focusing on feminist research methods and a postmodern epistemology. The applied qualitative method of online focus groups with participants from the global and academic level and from activists at local level is described. The identified results considering a framework for a FGHP are presented in Chapter 6, followed by a discussion of these findings and a methodological discussion (Chapter 7). Chapter 7 further entails recommendations for policymakers and researchers based on the results. The thesis ends with a conclusion and outlook (Chapter 8).

# Health Inequalities

Inequalities in health result from social inequality (Mackenbach, 2006; Marmot & Allen, 2014). While the term *equality* refers to equal treatment for everyone, the term *equity* acknowledges that there are structural factors which disadvantage certain populations and that their particular needs must be addressed. Accordingly, health and gender inequities are socially constructed differences which are avoidable and unfair (Heise et al., 2019). Equity comprises the fair allocation of resources to ensure the same point of departure for everyone. Hence, equity is a prerequisite to achieve equality, the latter being the overarching objective (Shawky, 2021; UNFPA, 2005; WHO, 2019b). To address health inequalities requires the recognition of underlying social inequalities and their causes, i.e. the "systematically unequal distribution of power, prestige and resources among groups in society." (Solar & Irwin, 2010, p. 20). Power is a crucial concept considering inequality as its distribution in society decides over privileges and oppression (Solar & Irwin, 2010). Hierarchical structures manifest power relations in society, most notably "due to patriarchy, colonialism, capitalism, [and] neoliberalism" (Heidari & Doyle, 2020, p. 75). This makes health inequality a political issue. Only by structural change initiated at the political level can genuine equality (through equity) be achieved (Solar & Irwin, 2010).

## 2.1 Conceptual Framework for Action on the Social Determinants of Health

Individual health is shaped by the social determinants of health. As part of the Commission on Social Determinants of Health of the World Health Organization (WHO), Solar and Irwin (2010) elaborated a conceptual framework for the SDOH. This framework will be presented briefly.

H. Eger, *Feminist Global Health Policy*, BestMasters,
https://doi.org/10.1007/978-3-658-43497-7_2

The socioeconomic-political context is the starting point of the framework, including the aspects of governance, macroeconomic, social, and public policies, and culture and societal values (Solar & Irwin, 2010). By placing the socioeconomic-political context first, the authors emphasise that health inequities—and thus health—are strongly influenced by these macrolevel factors. The structural determinants, also referred to as social determinants of health inequities, are influenced by the macrolevel and not modifiable by individual behaviour. The socioeconomic-political context determines the allocation of resources, power, prestige, and discrimination in society, resulting in social stratification (Solar & Irwin, 2010). This stratification creates a social hierarchy. The distribution of power and resources is fundamental for the individual socioeconomic position in this social hierarchy and decides over privileges and oppression. Key structural determinants, which act as social stratifiers, are social class, gender, and race. Hence, they "configure the health opportunities of social groups based on their placement within hierarchies of power, prestige and access to resources" (Solar & Irwin, 2010, p. 30). Taking the example of gender, "girls and women suffer systematic discrimination in access to power, prestige and resources", causing gender inequality (Solar & Irwin, 2010, p. 33). Through these mechanisms gender influences the position in the social hierarchy.

In practice, reciprocal relations exist among the components of the model, with the path not always linear. For instance, the health status can influence the socioeconomic position which in turn can affect policies. However, structural determinants constitute the most important pathway to health and well-being (Solar & Irwin, 2010).

Social inequities influence health inequities. The more equal a society is, the healthier is its population (Dhatt & Pley, 2021; Wilkinson & Pickett, 2010). A social gradient is evident, indicating that adverse health outcomes are visible at every level of the social hierarchy and not solely affect the most marginalised (Solar & Irwin, 2010; Wilkinson & Pickett, 2010). The influence of the macrolevel shapes health and well-being even before birth and persists throughout life (Permanyer & Spijker, 2021). The resulting socioeconomic position further determines the intermediary factors, i.e. the social determinants of health (Solar & Irwin, 2010). Underlying social stratification leads to differential exposure, vulnerability, and consequences. Through these pathways, inequities influence individual health outcomes (Solar & Irwin, 2010; WHO, 2016). Intermediary determinants encompass material circumstances, behavioural and biological factors, psychosocial factors, and the health system. They have a direct impact on health. The health system is a determinant on its own right, as its structure impacts access, quality, availability, and affordability of healthcare (Solar & Irwin, 2010; WHO, 2019b).

Public health research often exclusively focuses on the intermediary determinants (e.g. Dhawan et al., 2021; Schwingshackl et al., 2017; Wu et al., 2017). While these directly affect health and well-being and improvements can enhance individual health outcomes, it is crucial to address the structural determinants as causes of health inequalities for a sustainable and systemic solution (Solar & Irwin, 2010).

## 2.2    Intersectionality

Intersectionality refers to the understanding that multiple factors, which determine discrimination and privileges, coexist, interact, and mutually reinforce one another. Historically, this concept was articulated by Black feminist scholars who recognised the double burden of sexism and racism faced by Black, Indigenous and People of Colour (BIPoC) women in the USA (e.g. Crenshaw, 1989; Hill Collins, 2019; hooks, 1982). The first wave of feminism—and those succeeding—was predominantly composed of white, middle-class women and neglected the multiple oppressions experienced by other women, particularly those related to race and class (Crenshaw, 1989; Davis, 1981; hooks, 1982). Intersectionality considers "multiple axis of oppression" (WHO, 2020, p. 18), which are not simply additive but rather create new complex structures of privileges and oppression. This understanding highlights the complexity of discrimination and the heterogeneity of individuals impacted (Carastathis, 2014; Davis, 1981; Tolhurst et al., 2012). Privileges and oppression are shaped by power dynamics, as described by Solar and Irwin (2010) in the SDOH framework. Intersectionality is about acknowledging these dynamics by "point[ing] to the workings of power relations in producing social inequalities and the social problems they engender." (Hill Collins, 2019, p. 46; Kapilashrami & Hankivsky, 2018). The concept reveals how gender, race, and class—shaped by the inherent asymmetrical power regimes in patriarchy/sexism, racism/colonialism, and classism/capitalism respectively—intersect and cause structural discrimination of the oppressed population (Butler, 1999; Heidari & Doyle, 2020; Hill Collins, 2019). By placing power at its centre, intersectionality is "the most valid approach to analyse social stratification as a whole" (Yuval-Davis, 2016, p. 369) and serves as a useful tool to analyse global health inequalities (Kapilashrami & Hankivsky, 2018). An intersectional approach aims to improve the situation for everyone by focusing on the most marginalised first (Crenshaw, 1989).

*Intersectional gender analysis*

Gender, race, and class are only a selection of multiple intersecting factors. They are considered in this thesis due to their relevance as structural determinants in the SDOH framework (Solar & Irwin, 2010). As previously noted, discriminating factors are not additive and should be examined holistically. From a research-pragmatic perspective, however, it may be necessary to reduce complexity in research. Therefore, an intersectional gender analysis focuses on gender "as it remains one of the most pervasive forms of inequalities and important causes of poor health outcomes" and considers the interlinkage with further determinants and its consequences (WHO, 2020, p. 18). Gender has to be regarded in relation to other categories as it constitutes only one aspect when examining discrimination (Springer et al., 2012). However, its profound embeddedness in power relations and structural inequalities provides a useful entry point for an intersectional analysis (Kantola & Lombardo, 2017; WHO, 2020). Intersectional gender analysis is an important concept to guide research about inequalities (WHO, 2020). This is predominantly true for global health, with gender being "one of the most influential determinants of health inequalities between and within countries." (Dhatt & Pley, 2021, p. 1165).

## 2.2.1 Gender, Race, Class

Accordingly, this research is guided by the intersection of the structural determinants gender, race, and class, with a particular focus on gender. Underlying each of these determinants is a specific power system that produces "structural foundations for social inequalities, for example, the racism of white supremacy, the class exploitation associated with capitalism, and the sexism inherent in patriarchy." (Hill Collins, 2019, p. 39). Sexism, racism, and classism are the mechanisms within a matrix of power, which upholds and manifests social inequalities. They are "embedded in political, social, and economic systems" (Nash, 2020, p. 43). Depending on their inherent ideology, a particular population group is considered inferior. This causes oppression and discrimination at the individual, institutional, and societal level (Parker & Aggleton, 2003; Scherr, 2016).

*Sexism* can be defined as the oppression and discrimination on the basis of sex and/or gender. It reinforces the superiority of the male sex (Glick & Fiske, 1997). Sexism upholds patriarchy. *Patriarchy* is the underlying power regime. It structures gender inequality by oppressing everyone who does not align to the dominant notion of masculinity—in the public as well as private domain (Cyba, 2010; Nash, 2020). Sexism can be regarded as the essential instrument for the patriarchal system. Hence, there exists an interdependence between sexism and patriarchy since patriarchy is the cause for sexism and sexism maintains patriarchy (Becker, 1999; Glick & Fiske, 1997).

*Racism* is the oppression and discrimination on the basis of race and ethnicity, which includes the ascription of alleged differences. It upholds the belief in white supremacy and the inferiority of others, thus creating power asymmetries based on racialised assumptions (Miles, 1991; UN, 1965).

*Classism* describes the oppression and discrimination on the basis of social class. Ostensible lower classes are perceived as inferior. Classism is engendered by capitalism and simultaneously manifests the capitalist system (Barone, 1999).

Consistent with the concept of intersectionality, the power regimes underlying gender, race, and class are interdependent and mutually reinforcing (Butler, 1999; Hill Collins, 2000; Roig, 2021). The resulting intersecting privileges and oppressions are a global phenomenon (Hill Collins, 2000). The next section presents the structural determinants and their relevance.

### *Gender*

The significance of gender for health equality has already been highlighted. To understand its outstanding impact, the concept of gender needs to be examined in more detail.

*Gender* is socially constructed. As such, it is not an intrinsic trait, but rather developed by society. It is a dynamic concept that alters depending on the cultural context. Hence, it is relational (Butler, 1999; Courtenay, 2000; Springer et al., 2012). Gender is often regarded as the counterpart to sex, i.e. cultural vs. biological aspects. Feminist researchers question this sharp distinction and argue that sex, mostly understood in binary terms, also relies on a sociocultural understanding (e.g. Butler, 1999; Phillips, 2005). Moreover, a sharp distinction between sex and gender is not possible as external (socially influenced) triggers can lead to embodiment and biological changes (Heise et al., 2019; Springer et al., 2012; Williams et al., 2021). The interconnectedness of sex and gender and their influence on health must be recognised. In health research in particular, sex-disaggregated (binary) data often accounts as considering gender—a major shortcoming. Additionally, gender is often equalled with the inclusion of women. A thorough comprehension of gender encompasses *all* genders, irrespective of binary boundaries (Courtenay, 2000; Phillips, 2005). A holistic understanding of gender is integral to reduce gender and global health inequality.

The concept of gender in society is shaped by context-specific gender norms, gender roles, and gender relations (WHO, 2016). *Gender norms* comprise the socially influenced beliefs about people of all genders in society, in particular concerning men and women. They are the unspoken "social rules and expectations that keep the gender system intact." (Cislaghi & Heise, 2020, p. 410; WHO, 2016). Gender norms manifest through socialisation, which begins before birth. As soon as the sex of the unborn child is known, respective gender-related expectations are evoked, which become increasingly pronounced during adolescence (John et al., 2017; Mesman & Groeneveld, 2018). Hierarchical power relations shape these norms, which are embedded and reproduced in institutions. Institutionalisation and socialisation influence the individual behaviour and social interaction (Cislaghi & Heise, 2020; Heise et al., 2019). Due to the deep entrenchment of gender norms in society, they are very persistent. Nonetheless, as they are socially constituted, they can be challenged and changed (Gupta et al., 2019; Heise et al., 2019).

The perception of gender norms strongly influences gender roles and gender relations. *Gender roles* are defined as the expectations society places on men, women, and gender minorities (WHO, 2016). Culturally constructed notions of femininity and masculinity shape the anticipated behaviour. By conforming to these roles, gender stereotypes are reinforced (Courtenay, 2000). *Gender relations* are the resulting hierarchical relations between the different genders (WHO, 2016). The internalisation of gender norms manifests patriarchy. Patriarchy relies on these mechanisms to uphold the power asymmetry in favour of hegemonic masculinity and to the disadvantage of non-conforming genders (Connell, 1990; Courtenay, 2000). Hegemonic masculinity is defined as the "socially dominant gender construction that subordinates femininities as well as other forms of masculinity" (Courtenay, 2000, p. 1388). This enables discrimination based on sexism.

Gender norms, roles, and relations impact health and well-being (e.g. Gupta et al., 2019; Hawkes & Buse, 2013). The hierarchical gender regime influences access to the healthcare system (CSDH, 2008). Conforming to gender norms can lead to risky health behaviour with adverse health outcomes for all genders (Hawkes & Buse, 2013; Weber et al., 2019). Research on the commercial determinants of health has revealed how the industry uses gender norms to promote certain products and behaviours leading to negative health impacts (Dhatt & Pley, 2021; Gupta et al., 2019).

Specific examples of the gendered impact on health are provided in Section 2.2.2. Gender inequality further affects other health-related determinants, such as access to education and employment—with lifelong (health) impacts. The intersection of gender and other social stratifiers creates complex hierarchical relations that dictate privileges and discrimination. The determinants of race and class are examined below.

*Race*

Race, like gender, is a social and not a biological category. Both determinants are socially constructed and context-specific (Miles, 1991; Roig, 2021; Yam et al., 2021). Artificial distinctions based on race (and gender) have been invented as a justification for discriminating behaviour—i.e. racism (Lugones, 2016). The intersection of racism and sexism becomes apparent when looking at history: The notion of binary gender norms and hegemonic masculinity were exported through Western colonialism (hooks, 1982; Lugones, 2016; Williams et al., 2021). Racism is inherent in colonialism, since the latter is based on the profoundly unequal power regime of white (male) supremacy (Connell, 1990). Hence, during the time of slavery, it was BIPoC women who suffered most from the intersection of racism and sexism, with implications still visible today (Davis, 1981; hooks, 1982). Besides sexism, colonialism was closely intertwined with capitalism. It was capitalist intentions that fuelled colonialism. The exploitation of resources, raw materials, cheap labour, and the people in the colonies was driven by capitalist aspirations and led to increasing global inequality. Racism served as a justification for this exploitation (Miles, 1991). As BIPoC were regarded as inferior, their exploitation was accepted and even advocated. The effects are still evident today (Lessenich, 2018). The World Inequality Report 2022 highlights that "economic development in the 20th and 21st century is still based on the depletion of global resources and the use of extensive, cheap manpower in low-income countries." (Chancel et al., 2021, p. 173). In racialised societies, racism is also linked to classism. People belonging to racialised minorities often have a lower social status than the majority population. This intersecting inequity increases the risk of diseases (Noonan et al., 2016; Rommel et al., 2015). The negative impact of hierarchical power relations on health became particularly evident during the Covid-19 pandemic, when marginalised people were more affected by the disease and less considered in pandemic response measures (Büyüm et al., 2020).

Global health itself is deeply colonial. With its roots in colonial medicine, a Western understanding of medicine and health was applied universally, suppressing other kinds of knowledge (Affun-Adegbulu & Adegbulu, 2020; Yam et al., 2021). This colonial legacy is still apparent today. Colonialism has merely been replaced by coloniality, which implies "[w]hereas formal colonialism certainly ended, the political, economic, and cultural relations that characterized colonialism have not." (Hill Collins, 2019, p. 110; Affun-Adegbulu & Adegbulu, 2020). The consequences are evident: The majority of global health institutions are located in countries in the

Global North.[1] Epistemology, i.e. what counts as knowledge, as well as terminology, are dominated by the USA and Europe (Khan et al., 2022). Corresponding authors and scientific journals related to these regions are preferred. White supremacy within global health causes a global divide, disadvantaging the global majority population (Abimbola & Pai, 2020; Büyüm et al., 2020). Because the system itself is hierarchical and unjust it will not be able to adequately address structural discrimination causing health inequality (Büyüm et al., 2020; Yam et al., 2021). Decolonising global health demands a systemic change focusing on social justice (Abimbola & Pai, 2020; Büyüm et al., 2020).

*Class*
Asymmetrical power relations in capitalism cause global inequalities. The hierarchy of a globalised economy creates structural discrimination (Petchesky, 2016; Roig, 2021). The capitalist economy relies on a hierarchical class system since the exploitation of lower social classes is a precondition for the prosperity of higher classes. This asymmetrical power distribution causes classism, the oppression of lower classes—within and between states (Barone, 1999).

As presented before, capitalism is linked to racism and sexism, with de Lima Costa's words (2016): "heteronormativity, capitalism and racial classifications are always already intertwined" (p. 50). Capitalism benefits from the colonial and racial world structure. States from the Global North can flourish on the expense of states from the Global South (Arruzza et al., 2019; Lessenich, 2018; Wallerstein, 1974). Classism disproportionately affects people suffering from racism and sexism—creating intersecting discriminatory experiences (Connell, 1990; Davis, 1981). The global economy is highly gendered. The discrimination of women in the workforce, including (unpaid) care work is the result of interlinked sexism and capitalism. Although capitalism relies on this work, it oppresses female labourers by not acknowledging their financial value—which implies economic exploitation (Arruzza et al., 2019; Nash, 2020). Health equality is threatened by the "deleterious—and racist, sexist—health impacts of global capitalism" (Petchesky, 2016, p. 147). Capitalism, and in particular neoliberalism, strongly impacts the healthcare system by reducing public service provision. This particularly concerns people who already face structural discrimination (Arruzza et al., 2019; Petchesky, 2016). Apart from that there are more direct health consequences. Precarious employment and poverty are health risk factors that are strongly gendered (Brinkmann et al. 2006;

---

[1] In this thesis, the terms Global North and Global South are used. They are capitalised to indicate that they are to be understood as designation and not geographically. However, it is acknowledged that these terms are also contested (e.g. Khan et al., 2022; Teixeira da Silva, 2021).

Rogers, 2006). Specific examples of health consequences will be given in the next chapter.

## 2.2.2    Implications for health and well-being

As social inequality generates health inequality, adverse health outcomes result from the embodiment of these inequalities. Heise and colleagues (2019) elaborated a framework of the gender system and health. It entails the pathways through which gender affects health outcomes and encompasses the intersection with further structural determinants. The framework starts with the biological sex. Even before birth, when the sex of the child is determined, the social production of gender begins within the gender system. Gender norms, roles, and relations—depicted above—reproduce the gender system in the private and public sphere. The individual is assigned to a gendered social position, depending on the intersection with further structural determinants. Heise and colleagues (2019) identified five gendered pathways to health through which this position determines individual health outcomes. The pathways are presented briefly. Specific examples of adverse health implications are illustrated subsequently.

The first pathway comprises gender-related differences in exposure. For instance, gender roles shape the labour choices of women and men, which are associated with different health risks. The second pathway is gendered health behaviour. "[H]azardous masculinities and toxic femininities" have harmful implications for the health of all genders (Heise et al. 2019, p. 2444). Gender also impacts access to healthcare, the third pathway. Gender norms and an asymmetrical power distribution can restrict accessibility and affordability for those oppressed in patriarchy. The fourth pathway portrays that the healthcare system itself is gender-biased. Gender stereotypes lead to unequal treatment. Moreover, the health workforce is highly gendered, leaving women in lower-paid positions although they comprise the majority of the workforce. A gender bias is equally evident in health research, institutions, and data collection, the fifth pathway. Drug development that ignores gender inequality can have detrimental health effects (Heise et al., 2019). This framework is similarly applicable to other structural determinants which shape social inequality, including race and class.

Examples of health inequality, resulting from gender, racial, and class inequities and inequality leading to adverse health outcomes, are numerous. The following section is intended to provide a condensed, structured overview.

*Healthcare system*

Consistent with the framework by Heise and colleagues (2019), Hay and colleagues (2019) endorse that "restrictive gender norms manifest in the health system and reflect and reinforce gender inequalities, compromising the health and wellbeing of patients and providers." (p. 2543). Societal assumptions about gender and related expectations—i.e. gender norms and relations—influence the delivery of health services (WHO, 2019b). The intersection of discriminating factors further limits access to healthcare. In particular, gender and racial minorities face restrictions and discrimination within the system (Dhatt & Pley, 2021; Hay et al., 2019). Those already marginalised experience further exclusion with negative health impacts (EIGE, 2021; Roig, 2021). Globally, healthcare systems have not effectively addressed (gender) inequality, but rather have exacerbated it (Courtenay, 2000; Hay et al., 2019). This becomes apparent when looking at the health workforce. The workforce is organised hierarchically (Dhatt & Pley, 2021; Hay et al., 2019; Sen, Govender, & El-Gamal, 2020). Although women comprise 70 % of the workforce, only 25 % of senior positions are occupied by women (WHO, 2019a). In the informal health and care sector it is mostly women who engage in unpaid work (e.g. Winker, 2015). Lower-paid and unpaid occupations lead to a lower socioeconomic position, causing an intersection of patriarchy and classism (Dhatt & Pley, 2021; Hay et al., 2019). The organisation of the health workforce is influenced by gender norms and roles. Sexual harassment towards female health workers highlights this structural discrimination (Dhatt & Pley, 2021; Hay et al., 2019; Sen, Govender, & El-Gamal, 2020). Gender equality within the health workforce would also benefit patients, since a higher proportion of female health workers is related to improved health outcomes (Dhatt & Pley, 2021; Hay et al., 2019). However, gender parity should not be the only objective. As the problem is systemic and involves the macrolevel, structural change at political level is needed with equity and equality at its core (Hay et al., 2019; Sen, Govender, & El-Gamal, 2020).

Power asymmetries are equally visible at the leadership level of global health organisations (Global Health 50/50, 2022; Newman et al., 2017). The impact of patriarchy on gender norms and roles affects these organisations because they are embedded in society (Newman et al., 2017). The dominance of hegemonic masculinity portrays leaders as male. This depiction relies on gender stereotypes. It depends on women taking over family and household work, which simultaneously leaves them with inferior professional positions and career opportunities than their male counterparts. Again, the intersection of patriarchy and capitalism is evident (Newman et al., 2017). The Global Health 50/50 collective examined diversity in global health leadership and concluded: "Male dominance in global health pervades" (Global Health 50/50, 2022, p. 29). But the lack of diversity goes beyond gender. Global Health 50/50 analysed the composition of board members of the 146 most influential global health organisations: 75 % of board members came from high-income countries (HICs) (the majority from the USA) and only 2.5 % from low-income countries (LICs). Women accounted for 40 % of the board seats. This number decreases to 9 % for women from low-and-middle-income countries (LMICs). One board member out of over 2000 defined as non-binary. The global divide is highlighted by the location of the headquarters, with 94 % of the global health organisations registered in a HIC (Global Health 50/50, 2022). These results emphasise the intersecting global power regimes of patriarchy, racism, and capitalism in global health. Wenham and Davies (2021) examined the consideration of gender at the WHO. The WHO is regarded as the "ministry of health at the global level" (McCoy & Hilson, 2009, p. 218). The authors identified that the responses of the WHO to health emergencies were not gender-inclusive. Ignoring the underlying structures that cause different exposures to health risks can be harmful. As the leading global health organisation, the WHO should serve as a best practice example (Wenham & Davies, 2021).

### *Health Research*

Health research is highly gender-biased and therefore identified as a gendered pathway to health by Heise and colleagues (2019). White men are regarded as the standard, to the disadvantage of everyone else (Courtenay, 2000; Dhatt & Pley, 2021; WHO, 2019b). This is of particular concern regarding clinical trials. Until the 1990s, only men (mostly white) where included in clinical trials for pharmaceutical drug development. The main reasons for excluding women were the more complicated conditions related to the hormonal cycle and the risk of pregnancy (Benjeaa & Geysels, 2020; Liu & DiPietro, 2016).

Yet these factors are the reality of women's everyday lives—hence there is an even greater demand to include them in clinical trials. Focusing on men decreases the external validity of pharmaceuticals. Neglecting different circumstances has severe health implications. Medication that is not tested on the target population can result in overdosage and harmful side effects (Benjeaa & Geysels, 2020; Dhatt & Pley, 2021; Liu & DiPietro Mager, 2016). The consequences of male dominance in clinical trials are still apparent today. Men are regarded as the norm. Old pharmaceuticals that were only tested on the male population before market access continue to be prescribed (Benjeaa & Geysels, 2020; Liu & DiPietro, 2016).

Besides drug development, a gender bias is visible in the diagnosis and treatment of diseases. The most prominent example is cardiovascular disease. Medical students are taught the *typical* symptoms—which are only typical for men, while symptoms common in women are referred to as *atypical*. This androcentric perception is the result of patriarchy. Such misconceptions can lead to delayed treatment—followed by the danger of medication overdose (Canto et al., 2012; WHO, 2019b).

Overcoming this gender bias requires a focus on gender instead of sex, i.e. the social and structural factors that influence health, risk factors, compliance and therapeutic success. The demand for sex-disaggregated data, mostly relying on a heteronormative understanding, is insufficient (Williams et al., 2021). Another shortcoming of health research is its emphasis on quantitative data. While this is indisputably an essential aspect of research, the significance of qualitative insights should not be undervalued. In particular with regard to gender and intersectionality, an exclusive reliance on standardised statistics is inadequate as it neglects lived experiences and marginalised populations (Gupta et al., 2019; Heidari & Doyle, 2020). Health research must recognise power hierarchies. An intersectional understanding is crucial. Besides gender, a racial bias is evident in health research, negatively affecting the diagnosis and treatment of non-white people (Centola et al. 2021). With the increase of artificial intelligence in healthcare, bias in health research could become even more problematic because the software is influenced by underlying perceptions of society (Dhatt & Pley, 2021).

### *Sexual and reproductive health and rights*
Sexual and reproductive health and rights (SRHR) are pivotal for the achievement of equality and health and well-being for all. SRHR are composed of sexual rights, human rights, reproductive rights, sexual health, and reproductive health (Starrs et al., 2018). The realisation of SRHR is anchored in the Sustainable Development Goals (SDGs) and was first manifested at the International Conference on Population and Development in Cairo in 1994.[2] Starrs and colleagues (2018) have elaborated an updated, comprehensive definition of SRHR based on the WHO definition of health (WHO, 1946):

> Sexual and reproductive health is a state of physical, emotional, mental, and social wellbeing in relation to all aspects of sexuality and reproduction, not merely the absence of disease, dysfunction, or infirmity. [...] All individuals have a right to make decisions governing their bodies and to access services that support that right. Achievement of sexual and reproductive health relies on the realisation of sexual and reproductive rights, which are based on the human rights [...] (Starrs et al., 2018, p. 2646)

The authors emphasise that health services must be accessible, available, acceptable and of adequate quality. SRHR are strongly linked to aspects of autonomy

---

[2] More details on political endeavours are presented in Section 3.1.

and choice. This implies decisions about marriage and children, free sexuality including pleasure, access to resources and information, and a non-discriminatory environment (Starrs et al., 2018). Starrs and colleagues (2018) identified seven components of SRHR: gender-based violence (GBV), sexually-transmitted infections (STIs, including HIV/Aids), contraception, maternal and newborn health, abortion, infertility, and reproductive cancers. Achieving SRHR universally requires action beyond the health sector.

As SRHR are human rights, they are closely related to "power, politics, and patriarchy" (Gilmore & Khosla, 2020). The power imbalance causing gender inequity restrict SRHR (EIGE, 2021). Patriarchy influences prevailing gender norms regarding sexuality (Gilmore & Khosla, 2020). Considering this structural foundation, the political sphere plays an important part. Laws and policies determine the provision of and access to healthcare and reproductive services (Dhatt & Pley, 2021; Gilmore & Khosla, 2020). They are crucial for the fulfilment of SRHR but at the same time can severely restrict them. The recent overturn of *Roe v. Wade* in the USA is a prominent example. Political decisions concerning SRHR also have global consequences. For instance, the USA is a major donor in global health, but funding is generally restricted when it comes to SRHR and abortion in particular (Starrs et al., 2018). This directly impacts the health of women and gender minorities. Furthermore, the political level influences the society and its perception (Dhatt & Pley, 2021). SRHR concern everyone—also men—but once again, it is the marginalised who are most affected by unmet needs (Starrs et al., 2018). In patriarchy this includes everyone concerned by gender inequality. Hence, the fulfilment of SRHR is a profound feminist issue (Lunz, 2022). The interlinkage with further factors creates additional barriers towards the realisation of SRHR. For example, poverty and lack of education restrict individual autonomy (Starrs et al., 2018).

SRHR highlight the importance of an intersectional perspective. Reproductive rights are closely related to gender, race, and class. Capitalist interests influence reproduction. Depending on race and class, reproduction is either approved or discouraged (Hill Collins, 2000, 2019). The history of birth control and contraceptives roots back to slavery in the USA and is thus embedded in racism, classism, and sexism (Lunz, 2022; Roig, 2021; Ross & Solinger, 2017).[3] Capitalist aspirations endorsed a high birth rate among enslaved Black women—more children meant more unpaid labourers. This changed with the end of slavery. Eugenic ideology aimed for more white children. Hence, white women were denied terminating pregnancies while BIPoC women were forcibly sterilised. Poor women were also not

---

[3] Most research on racist and sexist intersections considering reproduction are conducted in the USA due to its (racial) history. Therefore, the presented examples refer to this context.

supposed to have many children as they were regarded as inferior by society and thus a burden to the welfare state (Davis, 1981; hooks, 1982; Ross & Solinger, 2017). The intersection of sexism, racism, and classism enforced social inequality and seriously restricted the realisation of SRHR. Reproduction was used as an instrument to control (BIPoC) women's bodies. Policies undermining access to SRHR healthcare point in the same direction today and provide the state with power over sexuality and bodily autonomy—mostly ignoring the fact that what is criminalised by policy continues illegally, with severe health risks attached (Connell, 1990).

To emphasise the existence of multiple power asymmetries and their influence on SRHR, the term *Reproductive justice* was developed (Ross & Solinger, 2017). This term combines aspects of reproductive rights and social justice. Reproductive justice considers underlying power relations since focusing only on legal rights is not sufficient. Justice includes further (social) changes according to individual needs. For example, access to SRHR is influenced by several determinants that are not equally addressed by legal change. Acknowledging intersectionality is central to reproductive justice. The term was introduced by BIPoC women in the 1990 s as resistance to dominant paradigms by white feminists. The latter focused on the right to abortion and the importance of individual choice, disregarding that BIPoC women faced structural discrimination concerning the right to reproduce and access barriers beyond the legal scope. Reproductive justice recognises inherent power regimes and the complexity of SRHR (Ross & Solinger, 2017). It "requires free, universal, not-for-profit health care, as well as the end of racist, eugenicist practices in the medical profession." (Arruzza et al., 2019, p. 14). To achieve reproductive justice, bodily autonomy is crucial. Globally, great unmet needs for modern contraceptives prevail. The latter implies contraception that is safe, efficient, and affordable. Hereby, policies play an integral role. Equally important is social change to address cultural barriers. The belief that contraception is a woman's responsibility is widespread and prevents men from getting involved (Starrs et al., 2018).

Another integral part of SRHR is abortion. Abortions occur globally. The right to abortion is highly dependent on policies and laws and influenced by gender norms (Starrs et al., 2018; WHO, 2019b). Unsafe abortions result from restrictive policies as well as from stigmatisation and discrimination in society. They pose a major threat to global health with detrimental health consequences for the mother and child—even resulting in death. Restricting access to safe abortion is hence a result of patriarchy. Safe abortion, which is not stigmatised by society or medical personnel, poses fewer health risks than delivery (Dhatt & Pley, 2021; Starrs et al., 2018). Restricted access to abortion causes adverse health effects, directly and indirectly. The Turnaway Study, a longitudinal study, examined the effects of being denied an abortion in the USA (Miller et al. 2020a). Women who had to proceed their pregnancy faced more severe health impacts, including life-threatening conditions, than women who underwent abortion. They also faced high financial strains, often related to raising the child alone (Miller et al. 2020a, b). The provision, accessibility, and affordability of safe abortions is crucial for realising SRHR.

Maternal and infant health are components of SRHR and closely linked to gender equality (Klugman et al., 2019). In the past, maternal and infant mortality has been considerably reduced worldwide. However, since the majority of these deaths is preventable, further efforts are needed. A global divide is evident. Maternal and infant mortality is significantly higher in LMICs than in HICs (Dhatt & Pley, 2021; Starrs et al., 2018). Klugman and colleagues (2019) identified a correlation between a higher score on the Women, Peace and Security Index and a reduction of death rates. The researchers "confirm significant positive associations between women's inclusion, justice, and security and maternal and infant mortality rates" (Klugman et al., 2019, p. 6). Death is the most extreme consequence of health inequities, but it begins with differences in morbidity and well-being. In addition to the global disparity between HICs and LMICs, maternal health is highly influenced by intersecting factors (EIGE, 2021). Marginalised communities are more exposed to health risks. Racial inequities amplify health inequalities. In the USA, pre-term births are 49 % more prevalent in Black women than non-Black women (March of Dimes, 2019). Racial discrimination also affects the health and lives of Black pregnant women in the United Kingdom. They have maternal mortality rates more than four times higher than white women (Knight et al. 2021). A systematic review and meta-analysis by van Daalen and colleagues (2022) confirms that racial discrimination leads to adverse pregnancy outcomes.

Diseases like STIs, Aids and cervical cancer highlight the direct health consequences of unmet SRHR. Prevention and treatment of cervical cancer intersect with class and race. Globally, far more women die in LMICs from cervical cancer, although it is preventable and treatable. Even within HICs, women from lower classes are more vulnerable (Dhatt & Pley, 2021; Starrs et al., 2018). The realisation of SRHR are especially important for adolescents as it determines their further life and health (Starrs et al., 2018). However, due to cultural and societal norms resulting from gender inequality, young women are particularly vulnerable to STIs and HIV/ Aids (Dhatt & Pley, 2021).

### *Gender-based violence*
GBV is one component of SRHR. Because it is the most extreme form of discrimination against women and gender minorities, it is examined in detail in this section. Starrs and colleagues (2018) define GBV as

any act of violence that is inflicted upon an individual because of his or her gender or sexual orientation [...] [it] encompasses harmful practices, such as child marriage, sex trafficking, honour killings, sex-selective abortion, female genital mutilation, and sexual harassment and abuse. (Starrs et al., 2018, p. 2652–2653)

GBV includes physical, sexual, and psychological violence (Sardinha et al., 2022; Starrs et al., 2018). A throughout assessment of GBV is difficult due to data limitations, in particular regarding psychological violence (EIGE, 2021; Sardinha et al., 2022). Research conducted by Sardinha and colleagues (2022) identified that in 2018 27 % "of ever-partnered women aged 15–49 years are estimated to have experienced physical or sexual, or both, intimate partner violence at least once in their lifetime" (p. 807–808). The authors emphasise that GBV is a global phenomenon. Although regional differences are evident, its prevalence is unacceptably high worldwide. LMICs and regions affected by conflict have a higher prevalence (Sardinha et al., 2022). This data was collected prior to the Covid-19 pandemic, which likely exacerbated the situation. GBV can result in death. Femicides, "the intentional murder of women and girls because of their gender" (UN, 2015a, Art 2), are the most severe manifestation of gender inequality. In 2020 an estimated 47,000 women and girls were killed globally by a close family member (UNODC, 2021). The overwhelming majority of GBV, particularly sexual violence, is committed by a male (ex-)partner (Dhatt & Pley, 2021; Starrs et al., 2018). Harmful notions of masculinity, evolving in patriarchy, endorse GBV. Violent behaviour is perceived as masculine and encouraged (hooks, 1982). Racist and classist discrimination enforce this deeply sexist conduct (Arruzza et al., 2019). Harmful practices, e.g. sex trafficking and female genital mutilation, are justified by persistent gender norms (Dhatt & Pley, 2021). Power asymmetries inherent in patriarchy are most profoundly revealed in GBV.

GBV is a major threat to health. Direct physical consequences encompass injuries or even death, STIs, and complications related to pregnancy. The impacts on mental health are devastating and oftentimes last a lifetime (Starrs et al., 2018; WHO, 2019b). Stigmatisation and discrimination, resulting from gender norms, can restrict access to healthcare, preventing individuals from receiving appropriate diagnosis and treatment (WHO, 2019b).

### Men's health

Recognising that gender inequality affects all genders, men also face particular health consequences (Courtenay, 2000; Dhatt & Pley, 2021). Research on the impact of patriarchy on men's health has long been neglected because gender is often regarded as synonym for women. However, underlying power regimes influence men's behaviour. Gender norms and gendered beliefs about health manifest hegemonic masculinity by presenting men as strong and dominant. By adhering to these gender roles, the patriarchal system is reinforced (Courtenay, 2000). This causes adverse health outcomes for men. Health-promoting behaviour connotes femininity in society, with the result that males tend to engage in health-risky behaviour (Courtenay, 2000). It is important not to regard men as a homogenous group. The intersection of social stratifiers, like race and class, creates different forms of privileges and discrimination among men as well.

As presented above, a distinction on the basis of sex is not sufficient. Rather, it is more adequate to consider the influence of hegemonic masculinity and gender inequity. Men who do not conform to hegemonic masculinity and heteronormativity are considerably more oppressed in patriarchy (Courtenay, 2000; Dhatt & Pley, 2021). Hence, it is not the male sex, but gendered behaviour resulting from social pressure to conform to hegemonic masculinity, that poses a health risk—consistent with the second gendered pathway to health according to Heise and colleagues' framework (Courtenay, 2000; Heise et al., 2019). Unhealthy behaviour causes negative health outcomes. Men tend to eat more unhealthy food, consume more alcohol and tobacco, and engage in more risky behaviour, for example resulting in deadly traffic accidents (Dhatt & Pley, 2021; WHO, 2019b). They also have higher morbidity and mortality rates for a range of diseases, e.g. tuberculosis and diabetes, often related to individual health factors (Dhatt & Pley, 2021). Regarding sexual and reproductive health, men are less likely to get tested for STIs and adhere to treatment, due to prevailing gender norms (Starrs et al., 2018). Work-related accidents occur disproportionately often in men, particularly in lower social classes, highlighting the intersection with classism (DGUV, 2021). Accordingly, hegemonic masculinity and patriarchy negatively affect the health of all genders.

### Health of transgender people

Research about the health of transgender people is scarce and mostly conducted in the USA.[4] The global size of the transgender population is unknown and difficult to examine. However, transgender people are present all over the world and include millions of people in absolute numbers, even if they represent only a small percentage of the total population (Reisner et al., 2016; Winter et al., 2016). Considering the health of transgender people, stigma and discrimination impose major barriers to good health and well-being (Reisner et al., 2016; Starrs et al., 2018;

---

[4] As the focus in this paper is on gender, research concerning sexuality and intersex people is not included.

Winter et al., 2016). The intersection with multiple determinants of health, influenced by stigma, impact negative health outcomes. For instance, transgender people lack access to education and employment opportunities in many parts of the world, which causes them to engage in precarious work (Winter et al., 2016). They frequently face violence and are denied basic human rights (Reisner et al., 2016). Discrimination of transgender people in society restricts their access to healthcare. Stigma is also prevalent among health workers, who lack knowledge and awareness about the needs of transgender people (Starrs et al., 2018). Precarious living and working conditions and the simultaneous lack of access to healthcare services exacerbate health outcomes. Transgender people have an increased risk for STIs and HIV. Adverse mental health constitutes a major burden (Reisner et al., 2016; Winter et al., 2016). The intersection of gender, race, and class aggravates health outcomes, e.g. transgender BIPoC or those living in poverty experience worse consequences (Winter et al., 2016).

Due to the oppression of the transgender population in society, their need for medical care is even greater, while at the same time discrimination causes restricted healthcare access.

### *Mental health*

Mental health can be regarded as a cross-cutting issue. The adverse health outcomes illustrated above are likely to deteriorate the mental health of the affected populations. Some examples have already been given in the respective sections. Structural discrimination resulting from power asymmetries is itself a risk factor for adverse mental health. Bracke and colleagues (2020) analysed the relation between gender equality and mental health. Gender-unequal countries face a higher burden of negative psychological health, particularly affecting the oppressed population. Improvements concerning gender equality would hence benefit everyone (Bracke et al., 2020). Socially constructed gender norms inherent in patriarchy constitute a burden with negative consequences. Zhou and colleagues (2018) identified that work-family conflicts lead to worse mental health outcomes in full-employed females in China. Due to prevailing gender roles, they are still responsible for care and household work, in addition to working full-time. Gender norms also pose a risk to men's mental health. Societal pressure caused by hegemonic masculinity and heteronormativity increases suicidal ideation in men while it prevents them from seeking help (King et al., 2020). Intersectionality is crucial to consider with regard to mental health. If multiple experiences of discrimination persist, the effects on psychological well-being are even worse. Discrimination, as well as poverty, creates stress with long-lasting consequences (Heise et al., 2019). Research confirms that racial discrimination leads to adverse mental health implications, with depression being the most frequent outcome (Kluge et al., 2020; Paradies et al., 2015; Williams, 2018). The same accounts for classism. Lower social classes are associated with worse mental health (Meyer et al., 2014). Lampert and colleagues (2018) examined this relation for children in Germany. They identified a social gradient regarding mental health, confirming negative consequences for lower classes.

The health consequences of racism and classism have already been included in the examples on gender inequality. Their significance as an independent risk factor for health and well-being will be briefly presented.

### Racism

Race, a social construct, "is less a risk factor itself than a marker of risk for racism-related exposures" (Ford & Airhihenbuwa, 2010, p. S33). Power hierarchies responsible for racial discrimination cause health inequalities. Hence, racism is a threat to health and well-being. In a literature review Noonan and colleagues (2016) identified that Black Americans have the worst health outcomes in the USA for all health outcomes examined. The intersection of racism with further determinants exacerbates the situation. Black people represent the poorest population group in the USA, resulting from structural discrimination. Poverty is a main health risk factor—thus aggravating adverse health outcomes. The intersection of discriminatory experiences faced by BIPoC women leaves them particularly vulnerable (Noonan et al., 2016). Racism also restricts access to healthcare services (Kluge et al., 2020; Williams, 2018). Racist discrimination causes health workers and society to believe harmful stereotypes, such as the widespread belief that Black people feel less pain (Affun-Adegbulu & Adegbulu, 2020). This has negative health consequences and drives diseases. Racist and colonialist attitudes were also visible during the Covid-19 pandemic. States in the Global South did not get access to lifesaving vaccines. The severe vaccine inequity was created by the Global North—and continues today. At the same time, success in pandemic responses by the Global South were questioned or disregarded on account of persisting colonial mentality (Büyüm et al., 2020).

### Classism

Individual health and well-being are strongly influenced by the conditions in which people work and live. This indicates that social class is of great relevance. The economic resources of an individual and society as a whole impact health outcomes as they decide over material, social, and psychological resources (Lundberg et al., 2016). Capitalism increases class inequalities and hence health inequalities (Scambler, 2019). As stated before, poverty itself is a major health risk factor. In capitalist societies, social class is related to education and employment, which profoundly impact health. Unemployment as well as precarious employment are known to neg-atively affect health (Brinkmann et al. 2006; Wilkinson & Marmot, 2004). The influence of classism on health can be examined on two levels, nationally within states and globally between states.

Lower income levels negatively affect health outcomes (Lundberg et al., 2016). However, income inequalities within countries adversely impact the whole society. Social stress prevalent in inegalitarian countries influence physical as well as mental health. Adverse consequences are visible on each level of society, creating a social gradient (Wilkinson & Marmot, 2004; Wilkinson & Pickett, 2010). The lower the social class, the higher the risk factors. This is due to socio-environmental factors and individual behaviour—which in turn is influenced by surrounding conditions (Lam-pert et al., 2018). Lampert and colleagues (2019) identified a significant difference in mortality and life expectancy depending on social class in Germany. A lower class implied a lower life expectancy and earlier mortality (Lampert, Hoebel, & Kroll, 2019). These disparities are already evident in children. The authors con-firmed that health inequalities based on social class exist among a social gradient (Lampert, Hoebel, Kuntz, et al., 2019). Classism increases the risk for a variety of diseases, e.g. cardiovascular diseases (Lampert et al., 2018). Self-perceived health of individuals from lower classes is equally lower (Hu et al., 2021; Stiftung Gesund-heitswissen, 2020). Coping and resilience mechanisms are less pronounced, as well as health awareness and health literacy, compared to higher social classes (Scam-bler, 2019; Stiftung Gesundheitswissen, 2020). Furthermore, social class influences access to healthcare. Restricted access can lead to a negative cycle by increasing both morbidity and poverty (McMaughan et al., 2020).

These class inequalities likewise affect health on a global scale. A significant association between gross domestic product (GDP) and health is confirmed (e.g. Safaei, 2012). For example, the GDP of a country is linked to its average mor-tality rate and life expectancy (Varkey et al., 2010). Health inequalities caused by classism can be reduced through social policies and protection schemes. The trend towards neoliberal economies—a market-focused approach—thus negatively affects the health of the population (Lundberg et al., 2016). Neo-colonial percep-tions forced LMICs in the 1980 s to adapt structural adjustment programmes based on a neoliberal model, resulting in a "low-income high-inequality trap" (Ray & Lin-den, 2018, p. 2). This intersection of colonialism and capitalism continues to impact the health of people living in the Global South to this day. The World Inequality Lab observes a stagnation of global spending on healthcare and proposes a global wealth tax as possible solution. The authors further notice an increase in health inequalities during the Covid-19 pandemic (Chancel et al., 2021). The global dis-parities revealed and intensified by the pandemic were mentioned before. In addition to racist and colonialist attitudes fostering global vaccine inequity, classism is an additional contributing factor.

The presented examples emphasise the political relevance. As Solar and Irwin (2010) highlight in the conceptual framework on the SDOH, the socioeconomic-political context shapes health (in)equities, which further affect health outcomes and equality. Thus, public and global health are always political (Safaei, 2012). Patriarchy, racism, and classism—and inherent social inequalities—result from the socioeconomic-political context. Previous research emphasises the reciprocal relation between democracy and gender equality (e.g. Markham & Foster, 2021; Safaei, 2012). Democracy and the fulfilment of human rights endorse gender equality and resulting health outcomes (Safaei, 2012). Likewise, gender equality is essential for democracy (Markham & Foster, 2021). Democratic principles, like representation, participation, accountability, human rights, and transparency enhance equality. Hence, negative health impacts resulting from inequality can be reduced (Safaei, 2012). Threats to democracy, including authoritarianism, but also capitalism, negatively influence equality and therefore health outcomes (Arruzza et al., 2019).

Positively speaking, this implies that political action can create change with impact on the whole society (e.g. Lundberg et al., 2016; Noonan et al., 2016; Solar & Irwin, 2010).

# Political Endeavours and Opportunities

**3**

This chapter highlights selected political endeavours and future opportunities. Political commitment towards more equality, particularly gender equality, is visible across all levels. Multilateral platforms, such as the United Nations (UN), G7, African Union (AU), or European Union (EU), provide to a greater or lesser extent strategies targeting gender equality (e.g. AU, 2019; EC, 2020a, b; G7 Gender Equality Advisory Council, 2021, UN, 2015b). The same applies to several nation states. Policies promoting gender equality generally include SRHR and are crucial for global health equality. How these commitments will be translated into action remain to be seen. However, it is apparent that despite of recent progress, accelerated action is necessary to truly achieve global equality.

## 3.1  Action Towards Gender and Health Equality

The United Nations are the highest multilateral organ. In 2015, the member states of the UN agreed on the 2030 Agenda for Sustainable Development, encompassing 17 Sustainable Development Goals to be achieved by 2030. The premise of the SDGs, "Leave no one behind", indicates an emphasis on equality (UN, 2015b). Three SDGs are of major concern regarding a feminist global health policy: SDG 3, 5, and 10.

SDG 3 thematises the health of the world population and demands to "Ensure healthy lives and promote well-being for all at all ages" (UN, 2015b, p. 14). It entails nine targets and four strategic approaches that serve to achieve the overall goal. Target SDG 3.8 addresses the implementation of Universal Health Coverage (UHC) while SDG 3.7 specifically mentions universal access to reproductive and sexual health services. SRHR are also targeted within SDG 5, the goal to "Achieve gender equality and empower all women and girls" (UN, 2015b,

p. 14). SDG 5 further encompasses the termination of discrimination, violence, and harmful practices based on gender. To achieve gender equality, emphasis is put on participation, empowerment, equal rights, and leadership. The third relevant goal is SDG 10: "Reduce inequality within and among countries" (UN, 2015b). This goal aims for more social, economic, and political inclusion while eliminating discrimination. Political interference is perceived as particularly critical in reducing economic inequalities. Considering the SDGs, their interlinkage is frequently mentioned. In this respect, even more—if not all—SDGs are important for global equality. An intersectional perspective is helpful to understand interacting aspects of the SDGs that influence privilege and oppression (Heise et al., 2019).

However, global efforts to address gender equality are not new to the SDGs. They have a long history, reaching back to at least four UN world conferences on women between 1975 and 1995 (UN Women, 2022b).

The most important and well-known conference for gender equality was held in Beijing in 1995. It resulted in the Beijing Declaration and the Platform for Action, which are regarded as major policy contributions towards gender equality (Beijing Declaration and Platform for Action, 1995). Although the documents specifically mention gender, they refer only to women and adopt a binary understanding of gender. The Beijing Declaration emphasises the rights of women and the need to end discrimination to achieve equality. The Platform for Action is the action-oriented companion document to implement the Declaration. It entails a holistic framework, covering twelve critical areas of concern—including health—and the related action needed. Both documents acknowledge the importance of an intersectional understanding due to the existence of "multiple barriers" (Beijing Declaration Art. 32, p. 4, p. 92). Another major focus of the Beijing conference was the establishment of gender mainstreaming as main strategy, i.e. the "systematic integration of a gender perspective at all levels" (CSDH, 2008, p. 149). The goals set forward in the Declaration and Platform for Action were meant to be achieved by the year 2000. Theoretically, the documents already contain all important aspects. The Platform for Action is genuinely comprehensive, providing key action steps, also for the health domain. However, 25 years after this milestone conference, the UN Commission on the Status of Women noted with concern that "no country has fully achieved gender equality and the empowerment of women and girls" (UN Women 2020, p. 3).

In addition to the world conferences on women, the UN adopted the Convention on the Elimination of All Forms of Discrimination against Women (CEDAW) in 1979. This convention is a pivotal document considering women's rights and equality. Although not mentioned once in the document, the convention is a major instrument against patriarchal structures. Furthermore, it includes an intersectional perspective by recognising different circumstances of women related to poverty and racism. To monitor the progress of CEDAW globally, the Committee on the Elimination of Discrimination against Women has been established.

The UN family comprises of several organisations and programmes (DGVN, n.d.; UN, 2021). Gender and health equality, despite being cross-cutting issues and affecting most entities, are particularly prominent in four UN organs: UN Women, United Nations Population Fund (UNFPA), United Nations Development Programme (UNDP), and WHO.

UN Women, short for United Nations Entity for Gender Equality and the Empowerment of Women, was established in 2010 explicitly to achieve gender equality worldwide (UN Women, 2022a). UNFPA is the specialised fund for sexual and reproductive health. Its mandate therefore inherently encompasses gender and health (UNFPA, 2022). UNDP focuses on global equality through the lens of development and poverty. Hereby, gender is also considered, manifested in UNDP's gender equality strategy. Health is another focal point, especially in relation to development (UNDP, 2022a; UNDP, 2022b).

The WHO is the UN specialised agency for health and regarded as central actor in global health. According to its Constitution, the objective is the "attainment by all peoples of the highest possible level of health" (WHO, 1946, p. 2, Art 1), which is considered as "one of the fundamental rights of every human being without distinction of race, religion, political belief, economic or social condition." (WHO, 1946, p. 1). This encompasses an intersectional commitment towards health equity and equality that is apparent throughout the entire work of the organisation. The endeavour by the WHO to achieve UHC reinforces this commitment. UHC entails that all people have access to healthcare according to their needs, without financial hardship (WHO, 2019b). The achievement of UHC is a major component of SDG 3 (UN, 2015b). However, criticism has been levelled regarding the focus on financial aspects and quantitative indicators to measure UHC. Concerns are raised that this narrows the scope to insurance coverage, neglecting the risks of private sector involvement and obstacles beyond financial difficulties. Measuring progress only by quantitative indicators is insufficient to detect inequities in access to healthcare (People's Health Movement et al., 2022). The primary health care (PHC) approach, brought forward by the International Conference on Primary Health Care 1978 in Alma Ata, recognises the complexity of health equality by prioritising a comprehensive basic care close to people's home, tailored to the specific needs of the population (Declaration of Alma-Ata, 1978, Art VI, VII). However, while this approach is pursued by the

WHO, it is criticised that PHC is merely subordinated to UHC (People's Health Movement et al., 2022).

Realising health for all requires equal opportunities free from discrimination. Hence, the WHO is an essential actor regarding health equality and further related equity and equality considerations. Efforts towards gender equality and improved health outcomes are apparent throughout the whole organisation, as well as commitments to reduce health inequalities originating from racial discrimination (WHO, 2001, 2021).

As key multilateral organisation, the UN and its organs play a major role regarding global equality. Decisive measures are already being taken, with the examples above only providing a selection. However, the full potential of the UN and related agencies is not yet realised (Allotey et al., 2019). Gender has to be understood comprehensively, not focusing solely on women and girls. The quantitative indicators to measure the SDGs are insufficient (Mair et al. 2017). Internally, the UN also faces gender-related problems, such as sexual harassment at the workplace. One recent extreme example is the sexual exploitation and abuse of women by WHO staff in the Democratic Republic of Kongo (Adepoju, 2022). Discriminatory structures within the UN system must be eliminated for the organisation to reach its global goals. Gender mainstreaming has not been implemented universally, partly resulting from a lack of accountability (Allotey et al., 2019; Mukhopadhyay, 2016). Strategies must be inherently intersectional, addressing the roots of inequalities. A feminist global health policy relies on an operational, powerful, restructured UN (Allotey et al., 2019).

Similar patterns can be observed in other multilateral organisations. Regarding the EU for example, gender equality is among its core values. The current gender equality strategy 2020—2025 as well as the EU Gender Action Plan III are comprehensive documents recognising the importance of an intersectional understanding (EC, 2020a, b). They likewise emphasise the need for gender mainstreaming across all institutions with the objective "to redistribute power, influence and resources in a fair and gender-equal way, tackling inequality, promoting fairness, and creating opportunity" (EC, 2020a, p. 16). The roots of gender inequalities are mentioned as well as further action to address these in accordance with SDG 5 (EC, 2020b). Reference is also made to the Council of Europe Convention on preventing and combating violence against women and domestic violence (Istanbul Convention). The Council of Europe comprises 46 member states, of which 35 have ratified the Convention. The Istanbul Convention focuses on violence against women and recognises underlying power hierarchies. This makes it a significant international treaty for women's rights. However, as with the UN, gender equality is typically understood with reference to women and girls.

Again, it is apparent that everything required for gender equality is present in theory. However, implementation is lacking. On global level, this is largely due to the dependence of multilateral organisations on their member states. These organisations are only as strong as their members. Finding a consensus between different interests—and implementing it accordingly—often proves difficult in reality.

## 3.2    Feminist Global Health Policy

Feminism today is not only about women, it encompasses a variety of aspects and "addresses structural injustice, social justice, and the future of the planet" (Goulimari, 2020, p. 2). Diverse strands of feminism highlight different issues. However, most feminist perspectives are based on intersectionality. They focus on the marginalised, linking various kinds of structural oppression in their analysis.

### Intersectional feminism
Intersectional feminism entails a holistic understanding of feminism. It recognises the significance of power hierarchies and resulting inequalities. While the focus is on eliminating patriarchy, all oppressing structures are fought against, including racism, colonialism, capitalism, and classism (Heidari & Doyle, 2020; Lunz, 2022). This implies that feminism also includes men, as they too can suffer from existing power asymmetries based on their individual position (Lunz, 2022). In this regard, Arruzza and colleagues (2019) describe feminism as "Standing for all who are exploited, dominated, and oppressed, it aims to become a source of hope for the whole human-ity. That is why we call it a *feminism for the 99 percent*." (Arruzza et al., 2019, p. 14, emphasis in original). Therefore, intersectional feminism is essentially decolonis-ing (Heidari & Doyle, 2020). Feminism is inherently political. It recognises the political significance because structural inequalities originate there (Connell, 1990; Rogers, 2006). According to Connell (1990), nation states are the "institutional-ization of power relations" (p. 520). Patriarchy is profoundly embedded in their system, as well as other forms of oppressing structures like classism and colonial-ism. In accordance with intersectionality, these power regimes influence each other and are interlinked, but at the same time they exist autonomously (Connell, 1990). In alignment with the framework on the SDOH by Solar and Irwin (2010), feminist approaches address the political level to generate social change. Feminism relies

on participation and the inclusion of civil society (Heidari & Doyle, 2020; Rogers, 2006).

### Towards a feminist global health policy

Williams and colleagues (2021) define health policy as "a collection of principles that have been created with the intent of guiding decisions specific to shaping health outcomes, broadly defined via the social determinants of health" (Williams et al., 2021, p. 1). A feminist global health policy focuses on the most disadvantaged first, acknowledging and challenging underlying power regimes (Davies et al., 2019; Rogers, 2006). According to the Centre for Feminist Foreign Policy (CFFP) a FGHP is

> about ensuring everyone has equal access to all aspects of health care [...] centering the needs of the most marginalised and actively contributing to overcome structural discrimination in all its forms. (CFFP, 2021, p. 1)

It considers the relation between health outcomes and power distribution and aims for equality by dismantling existing hierarchies. An intersectional feminist global health policy focuses on gender and the interlinkage with further structural determinants and their inherent asymmetrical power regimes. Based on a holistic, human rights approach, such a policy can mitigate health inequalities which derive from social inequalities (CFFP, 2021; Davies et al., 2019; Heidari & Doyle, 2020; Rogers, 2006).

A feminist approach to global health policy emphasises the power dimension. It highlights structural barriers emerging from the macrolevel that restrict equal health opportunities for all (CFFP, 2021; Rogers, 2006; Sen, Iyer, et al., 2020). Furthermore, intersectionality is fundamental for a FGHP (Davies et al., 2019). Since the focus is on asymmetrical power regimes, it is integral to understand the complexity of these structures and their effect on health. Sexism, racism, and classism—as well as further oppressing regimes—must be considered within the patriarchal system. This ensures a holistic comprehension of individual positions and health consequences (CFFP, 2021; Davies et al., 2019). Therefore, a FGHP demands a transformative system change, rather than isolated adjustments. By definition, this includes everyone—not only women or gender minorities. Accordingly, a feminist approach encompasses the whole health system, not merely specific issues.

In addition to being feminist, this approach comprises a global dimension. Globalisation aligns people worldwide. This also applies to health, with the Covid-19 pandemic demonstrating the most recent example—including for the failure of a global response. Global problems demand global solutions. As presented above, global health itself has a deeply colonialised history, with continuing implications. Unequal power relations persist worldwide and shape the health of people. A feminist global health policy provides an alternative by transforming the system towards equity and equality (Lunz, 2022). Therefore, a decolonial global framework can provide guidance to decision-makers and be adapted to specific contexts.

To dismantle power hierarchies and create equality, a FGHP depends on the inclusion of civil society. Only by involving activists and social movements, health equality can be achieved (Fulu et al., 2021). They are active on the ground and aware of the needs and social environment of the (marginalised) people. The empowerment of discriminated populations and their social, political, and economic participation is critical. Empowerment is identified as a protective health factor—for the individual as well as for society (Varkey et al., 2010). However, to enable participation, the right political preconditions must be in place. Especially health inequities need to be confronted from both sides—the political level and civil society (CSDH, 2008). Today, feminist movements in particular face massive resistance from right-wing, conservative and fundamentalist groups (Fulu et al., 2021). An enabling environment strengthens civil society and the agency of individuals. A feminist global health policy endeavours to generate this environment and to connect the political and social spheres.

# Research Interest and Research Question

According to the presented theoretical background, structural determinants shaped by the political context affect health and well-being. Key determinants influencing health inequity are gender, race, and class (Solar & Irwin, 2010). Grounded on the concept of intersectionality, inherent power regimes create structures of privilege and oppression that are interconnected and mutually reinforcing, causing individual experiences of discrimination. The resulting social position influences health (in)equity and affects health outcomes and equality (Kapilashrami & Hankivsky; Solar & Irwin, 2010). Previous work highlights that a FGHP is suitable to address these health inequalities by presenting an alternative approach to global health with a focus on mutuality, human rights, equity, and the most discriminated people first (CFFP, 2021; Davies et al., 2019). The potential of a feminist approach for health equality is hence highly relevant for public and global health. Likewise, the political foundation of this topic is of considerable importance for the field of political science and policy-making. Accordingly, research on feminist global health policy is an interdisciplinary endeavour providing valuable insights for both disciplines and the combined realm of global health policy.

Insightful research and information on the topic exist, presented in the previous chapters. However, as the topic is rather new, it lacks an action-oriented focus. In order not to remain an abstract construct, concrete and practical instructions are required. Further research is needed on what a feminist global health policy encompasses and how it can be adopted. This master's thesis is intended to address this research gap and to provide added value to the topic. In this regard, the following research question is examined:

H. Eger, *Feminist Global Health Policy*, BestMasters,
https://doi.org/10.1007/978-3-658-43497-7_4

**How can a feminist approach to global health policy be meaningfully implemented to reduce health inequalities?**

This research question is composed of two parts, with the main anticipated outcome being a framework for a feminist global health policy. This framework is intended, firstly, to establish principles and components of a FGHP. Secondly, guidance for the concrete implementation of a FGHP is to be provided. The intention is to ensure a link between the strategic, global level and an action-oriented, local level.

# Research Methodology 5

This chapter presents the research process and guiding principles upon which this thesis is based. The methodology is described extensively to enhance credibility and transferability of the results (Bryman, 2016; Tracy, 2010).

## 5.1 Research Design

Profound consideration of the research design is essential for the research question to be answered appropriately. The research design determines the quality of research and hence the results. It should be comprehensible and transparent to allow for traceability (Bryman, 2016).

### 5.1.1 Interdisciplinarity

This research is guided by an interdisciplinary approach. The subject of global health itself is inherently interdisciplinary and comprises a political dimension (Hanefeld & Fischer, 2021; Koplan et al., 2009). According to the widely recognised definition by Koplan and colleagues (2009),

> global health is an area for study, research, and practice that places a priority on improving health and achieving equity in health for all people worldwide. Global health emphasises transnational health issues, determinants, and solutions; involves many disciplines within and beyond the health sciences and promotes interdisciplinary collaboration (Koplan et al., 2009, p. 1995)

© The Author(s), under exclusive license to Springer Fachmedien Wiesbaden GmbH, part of Springer Nature 2023
H. Eger, *Feminist Global Health Policy*, BestMasters,
https://doi.org/10.1007/978-3-658-43497-7_5

As health inequalities persist globally, a holistic and systemic response that incorporates insights from multiple disciplines is crucial (Kivits et al., 2019). Addressing the social determinants of health in particular requires an interdisciplinary endeavour, considering the importance of the socioeconomic-political level in the framework by Solar and Irwin (2010). More specifically, research about global health policy should integrate public/global health and political science perspectives. Both disciplines are considered throughout this research at all stages. Aboelela and colleagues (2007) identify interdisciplinary research as present when theoretical frameworks, research design, and methodology are included from / common in both disciplines throughout the research. These components are considered in this thesis and referred to in detail below. Furthermore, interdisciplinary research is characterised by collaboration (Aboelela et al., 2007; Padberg, 2014). This aspect is incorporated in this study, highlighted in the sub-section *Participatory research*. The intersectional scope of the topic further emphasises an intrinsically interdisciplinary approach (Dill & Kohlman, 2012).

## 5.1.2  Feminist Research

Feminist research is applied in this project. This includes a strong emphasis on power regimes and knowledge production (Kaur & Nagaich, 2019). Feminist approaches acknowledge that research does not happen in a value-free, objective environment, but is rather shaped by existing power hierarchies and societal inequalities (Connell, 1990; McHugh, 2014). Knowledge presented as objective by traditional research is actually biased and influenced by social norms and dominating positions, including androcentric and colonial assumptions (Dill & Kohlman, 2012; Wigginton & Lafrance, 2019). By framing certain findings as knowledge and facts, while devaluing others as subjective, the Global North imposed—and continues to do so—its paradigms of knowledge and research (Hill Collins, 2019; Khan et al., 2022). Similarly, power asymmetries resulting from patriarchy are reproduced in research (Cook & Fonow, 2019). Feminist research aims to constitute an alternative. Considering intersectionality, it intends to foster social change and equality (McHugh, 2014). It recognises power regimes and focuses on structural discrimination. Hence, feminist research is action-oriented, emphasising participation and empowerment (Cook & Fonow, 2019; Kaur & Nagaich, 2019). The principles of objectivity and neutrality are challenged as research is always embedded in a social context. Objectification is avoided as well as the devaluation of subjective and individual experiences. Thus,

feminist research questions what counts as knowledge. It is inherently decolonising and seeks to terminate patriarchy (Cook & Fonow, 2019; McHugh, 2014;
Wigginton & Lafrance, 2019).

### Qualitative Research

Accordingly, qualitative research methods are generally better suited for feminist
approaches than quantitative research (Bryman, 2016; Kaur & Nagaich, 2019).[1]
Traditional research methods do not reflect on power regimes and follow standardised procedures—the standard usually being based on androcentric, colonialised
norms (Bryman, 2016; Wigginton & Lafrance, 2019). Participants are objectified
and exploited for the purpose of the research. Qualitative methods acknowledge individual experiences and consider the context and setting. They are typically based
on a post-positivist approach, i.e. dismissing the assumption that there is an objective, measurable truth to be uncovered and instead focusing on understanding a
socially constructed reality (Bryman, 2016). The objective of qualitative research
is not to generalise or standardise results but acknowledging the subjectivity of the
participants. Hence, it does not follow a predetermined structure. Regarding global
health, qualitative research is crucial to study the social determinants of health as
well as marginalised populations by listening to often unheard voices (CSDH, 2008;
Liamputtong & Rice, 2021). Furthermore, this approach is adequate when applying
an action focus and political lens (Bryman, 2016). Consequently, this project adopts
qualitative research methods to implement a feminist approach.

The choice of research methods is grounded in fundamental principles that
reflect on how the world is perceived and knowledge produced. The following
sections briefly present the ontology, epistemology, and methodology underlying
this research project, consistent with a feminist approach. However, a sharp distinction between these dimensions is not possible as they are intertwined and mutually
influencing (Maruska, 2017).

### Ontology

*Ontology* is understood as the researcher's understanding and perception of the
world. Considering the constructiveness of gender, race, and class, and resulting discrimination, this research is based on a critical, constructionist ontology.
It is assumed that the world is socially constructed through interaction. Existing

---

[1] However, this does not imply that all qualitative research is automatically feminist. The
acknowledgment of the depicted principles is decisive for (quantitative and qualitative)
research to qualify as feminist (Wigginton & Lafrance, 2019).

structures are questioned and challenged because they are considered as modifiable (Bryman, 2016; Maruska, 2017).

*Epistemology*

The choice of ontology further influences the epistemology this research is premised on. *Epistemology* is referred to as theory of knowledge. It reflects on how knowledge is produced and what counts as knowledge (Maruska, 2017). Such considerations highly affect the research process. Depending on the epistemological underpinning, certain methods are either preferred or regarded as insufficient (Bryman, 2016; McHugh, 2014). The production of knowledge, in global health and beyond, is highly colonial. The Global North dictates what qualifies as knowledge and imposes its perception on the rest of the world (Khan et al., 2022). Hence, epistemology is concerned with power and consequently a political matter (Hill Collins, 2019). Epistemological positions roughly range from positivist to post-positivist considerations, with multiple nuances in-between (Maruska, 2017). In feminist research, three major epistemologies have emerged: feminist empiricism, feminist standpoint, and postmodernism (Harding, 1987).

*Feminist empiricism* is most similar to traditional research, following a positivist approach to science and applying similar methods and principles (Wigginton & Lafrance, 2019). In contrast to traditional research, the feminist approach aims to eliminate "sexist and androcentric biases" (Harding, 1987, p. 182) by recognising and addressing prejudices throughout the research process. The two other feminist epistemologies differ significantly from feminist empiricism by distancing themselves from traditional research paradigms (McHugh, 2014; Wigginton & Lafrance, 2019).

*Feminist standpoint* theorists shift the focus from the researcher to the researched by emphasising the individual position. They believe in an external reality, which can be studied by taking the social context into account and acknowledging individual standpoint, experiences, and knowledge—of the researched as well as the researcher (Harding, 1987; McHugh, 2014; Wigginton & Lafrance, 2019). Considering intersectionality, more than one standpoint exists and needs to be recognised. This comprehension lies at the core of postmodernism (Harding, 1987; Maruska, 2017). However, the distinction between standpoint theory and postmodernism is not always straightforward (Maruska, 2017).

*Postmodernism* rejects the notion of an objective truth. Rather, reality is perceived as socially constructed and subjective (McHugh, 2014; Wigginton & Lafrance, 2019). This epistemological position is critical towards systemic theories that tend to provide extensive explanations (Gannon & Davies, 2012; Wigginton & Lafrance,

2019). It assumes that reality is relative, depending on the social and political context, which further shapes knowledge and experiences (Wigginton & Lafrance, 2019). Emphasis is put on power relations and their implications (Maruska, 2017; McHugh, 2014). Hence, "knowledge is contextual, historically situated, and discursively produced; [...] subjects are constituted within networks of power and knowledge." (Gannon & Davies, 2012, p. 79). As truth is socially constructed, multiple standpoints and contexts must be considered. This implies that science cannot be value-free, since it is always biased by the context and subjectivity of research participants and researchers (Maruska, 2017; McHugh, 2014). Postmodernist researchers therefore emphasise language and discourse (Cook & Fonow, 2019; Gannon & Davies, 2012).

This study is based on a postmodern epistemology, in line with a constructionist ontology. Intersectionality can be best researched by taking multiple standpoints into account. Furthermore, the social construction of the determinants gender, race, and class is well reflected in a postmodern approach. Postmodernism emphasises the social and political context as well as power relations, which are central to this research project.

### Methodology

The applied *methodology* depends on the epistemology. Methodology is understood as the way of engaging in research. This further influences the choice of methods (Cook & Fonow, 2019; Maruska, 2017). Maruska (2017) categorises methodologies as ranging from empiricist to interpretivist. The latter focuses on *understanding* as the main research objective (Bryman, 2016; Liamputtong & Rice, 2021). In line with a postmodern epistemology, this research project pursues an interpretivist methodology, by considering power and context (Maruska, 2017; Westkott, 2019). Furthermore, feminist research must be non-exploitative, regarding power distribution throughout the research process (McHugh, 2014). For this to be achieved, reflexivity should be integrated. This entails the acknowledgement of the researcher's individual position and of power hierarchies within the research, as these factors highly influence the results (Cook & Fonow, 2019; Gannon & Davies, 2012; Hill Collins, 2019). Reflexivity also promotes consciousness-raising, an important element emphasised by feminist researchers (McHugh, 2014; Westkott, 2019).

### Methods

Considering the choice of a constructionist ontology, postmodern epistemology, and interpretivist methodology, qualitative *methods* are applied in this research. The benefits of qualitative methods for feminist research have been presented above.

The focus on language and discourse as well as the emphasis on power highlighted by postmodernism can be best achieved with qualitative methods (McHugh, 2014). Consistent with the presented reflections, focus groups are employed as qualitative data collection tool, as portrayed in Section 5.2.

### 5.1.3   Participatory research

Participation is another major component of feminist research. An interactive, collaborative approach reduces hierarchies within the research process and places the participants at the centre (Cook & Fonow, 2019; Haig, 1999). Participation is particularly valuable regarding action-oriented research because the inclusion of participants facilitates the development of practicable recommendations (McHugh, 2014; Wright, 2021). Considering coloniality in global health and the urgent need to terminate it, participatory research is highly relevant to this field (Liamputtong & Rice, 2021). For health research in general, this approach is essential to study the social determinants of health, which are often overlooked in traditional biomedical research. However, participatory research became a popular catch phrase in public health. Therefore, it is crucial to ensure true participation (Wright, 2021). Guided by a postmodern epistemology, the choice of focus groups intends to enable an interactive, participatory research environment.

### 5.1.4   Quality criteria

Quality criteria serve to evaluate the research process. The choice of criteria is dependent on epistemology and methods (Kuckartz, 2016). While some researchers prefer to apply criteria common in quantitative research for qualitative studies, there exist several criteria for qualitative research. As this research project is based on feminist methods and a postmodern epistemology, specific criteria for qualitative research are perceived as more appropriate. Tracy (2010) identified eight universal criteria for qualitative research, which provide flexibility to be applicable to various qualitative projects. The present research is guided by these criteria. The first criterion is *worthy topic*, meaning that the chosen topic is relevant and timely. Given that the topic of feminist global health policy addresses persisting structural challenges and the results are intended to foster health equality, this criterion is considered to be met. The second criterion, *rich rigor*, is to be achieved by including a variety of perspectives in the focus groups and by acknowledging intersectionality. *Sincerity* is considered by reflexivity of the researcher as well as a transparent description of the process, which likewise enhances *credibility*. Feminist participatory methods also ensure multivocality and member reflection, as participants express their own perspectives and are invited to provide feedback on the results, which supports the criterion of credibility. Tracy (2010) further identifies *resonance* among the audience as a criterion, including transferability of results. Qualitative research should provide a *significant contribution*, theoretically, heuristically, practically, and methodologically. The topic and method of this thesis are chosen with regard to this aspect. Ethical considerations concerning the research process, depicted in Section 5.7, fit the *ethical* criterion. *Meaningful coherence*, the last criterion, describes the coherence between literature, research question, and results. It is to be fulfilled through the consideration of consistent ontology, epistemology, methodology and methods (Tracy, 2010). The evaluation of the quality criteria in this research is part of the methodological discussion in Section 7.2.

## 5.2    Data Collection Instrument

The data for this research project is obtained through focus groups. The choice of focus groups is consistent with a postmodern epistemology and interpretivist methodology and aligns with the principles of feminist research (Bryman, 2016; Wilkinson, 1999). The focus is on the participants instead of the researcher, reducing power asymmetries and the risk of objectification. The researcher mainly moderates the discussion and remains in the background (Bryman, 2016; Lamnek & Krell, 2016; Wilkinson, 1999). Exploitation criticised in traditional research is thus avoided. In contrast to interviews, emphasis is on interaction (Blatter et al., 2018; Kitzinger, 1995). As a result, participation is facilitated with the potential to gather new insights and produce knowledge (Stanley, 2016). In accordance with postmodernism, the social context is recognised in focus groups by taking different perspectives into account (Lamnek & Krell, 2016; Wilkinson, 1999).

The method of focus groups is common in health research (e.g. Tausch & Menold, 2015) as well as in political science (e.g. Blatter et al., 2018; Stanley, 2016). In particular, action-orientation and empowerment—inherently feminist principles—make it a convenient instrument for these disciplines. The participative element enables consciousness-raising and transformative results (Wilkinson, 1999). Kahan (2001) states that focus groups are specifically suitable for policy analysis and elaborating policy recommendations. By directly including the participants in the process, more meaningful policy outcomes emerge. The results should be made available for the participants to ensure true participation and avoid exploitation (Kahan, 2001).

Regarding the formalities of focus groups, there is no standard concerning the number of groups and participants required. The amount depends on the objective and principles of the research project as well as feasibility (Bryman, 2016). Group sizes of four to eight participants are common in the literature (Bryman, 2016; Kitzinger, 1995). Focus group discussions usually last one to two hours (Kitzinger, 1995; Tausch & Menold, 2015). In this research project, synchronous online focus groups are conducted. While it might be more difficult to create a comfortable atmosphere online and allow for extensive interaction, the use of audio-visual tools such as Zoom provides some advantages. The involvement of participants irrespective of their residence is possible at low cost and convenient for everyone concerned (Bryman, 2016; Lamnek & Krell, 2016). Regarding the global scope of this research, this is of major advantage.

*Intersectional gender analysis*
To comprehensively identify and address health inequalities and underlying power regimes, the selection of the right data collection instrument is crucial. The method of focus groups aligns with the directives of an intersectional gender analysis (Jhpiego, 2016; WHO, 2020). Ideally, research should be gender-transformative. Based on the toolkit by the WHO (2020) to incorporate intersectional gender analysis, this research project fulfils the criteria of gender-transformative research. First, the objective is to identify, address, and challenge health inequities. Hereby, particular focus is on power regimes and the structural dimension. Throughout the research process an intersectional gender lens is incorporated by using gender as entry point and recognising the interlinkage with race and class. As feminist and participatory research methods are applied, power is shifted to the people concerned. This implies the engagement of "relevant stakeholders" (WHO, 2020, p. 25). The action-oriented aim of identifying feasible recommendations to challenge and ultimately change existing (gendered) power relations has a genuinely transformative character. Consequently, the chosen data collection tool enables gender-transformative research with respect to an intersectional gender analysis.

## 5.3   Sampling Technique

The participants for the focus groups were recruited using purposive sampling. This non-random sampling method allows the researcher to choose participants according to the research objective and based on strategic assumptions (Bryman, 2016). Purposive sampling is a well-established technique for focus groups (Tausch & Menold, 2015). The sampling strategy applied in this research comprises of two levels. The first level refers to the context by deciding on different groups. The second level concerns the selection of participants within the respective groups (Bryman, 2016). Regarding the composition of groups, homogenous groups are preferred in the literature (Kahan, 2001; Lamnek & Krell, 2016). However, it is important to include different perspectives. Therefore, two or more homogenous groups that differ from each other should be included. Homogeneity here refers primarily to the thematic background of the participants. Other characteristics can be heterogeneous, for example the place of residence and age (Kahan, 2001; Lamnek & Krell, 2016).

*Inclusion and exclusion criteria*
In this study, three focus groups (FG1, FG2, FG3) were conducted. Consistent with the literature, participants from the same group showed homogenous interests. For the purposive sampling strategy, the following inclusion and exclusion criteria were adapted:

Inclusion in FG1 was based on affiliation with the strategic and/or academic level, i.e. universities, research institutions, UN organisations. As additional criterion, their work had to be linked to the global sphere and related to either global health, gender, feminism, intersectionality, or global inequalities. FG2 and FG3 comprised participants who were active at the local level, including members of civil society organisations, social movements, activists, and marginalised populations. Inclusion was considered if the participants' background was related to feminism, decolonialism, gender, health, inequalities, or intersectionality.

The remaining criteria were identical for all groups. Apart from the thematic background, diversity was intended. Purposive sampling was applied to ensure global reach. The objective was to include primarily participants from different parts of the Global South as representatives of the Majority World. Hence, region of residence or work served as inclusion criterion. Since the focus groups were conducted in English, only English-speaking participants could be included. Gender was not primarily an inclusion or exclusion factor because a feminist global health policy intends to be beneficial for everyone. However, attention was given to ensure that people who are discriminated against in patriarchy and by intersecting power regimes constituted the vast majority. Exclusion criteria were thus the lack of English knowledge, non-coherence with the topic, and affiliation with an already overrepresented region.

The objective of this purposive sampling strategy was to recruit the most appropriate composition with respect to the research question. The selection of the three focus groups was intended to link the global strategic-academic level with the local and action-focused level. By including different standpoints, the focus was on what is genuinely feasible and required by people on the ground, since action-orientation is an important aspect of policy framing.

### Sampling procedure

Based on the inclusion and exclusion criteria presented above, potential participants were identified. Potential participants were either known to the researcher through authorship or webinar keynotes on relevant topics, or they were found through extensive internet research on the subject, including affiliation to activist networks or organisations. A comprehensive list of potential participants was compiled, of which 33 people were contacted via e-mail. The first correspondence included a cover letter and a short graphic outline of the research project. A reminder was sent after two to three weeks. Two participants were referred by requested persons who could not attend and therefore forwarded the inquiry to colleagues.

### Participants

In total, 11 people participated in this study. FG1 comprised of six participants, FG2 of three and FG3 of two participants. Initially, two focus groups were planned. As one participant was not able to join due to technical issues, FG2 comprised of only three participants. However, this has turned out to be an advantage for the interaction and atmosphere. In order to establish a balance with the number of participants in FG1, and to enable participation for those who could not attend previously, it was decided to conduct a third focus group with three feminist activists. This also allowed for more perspectives to be included and extended findings. Eventually, one participant did not show up for FG3. However, this did not detract from the discussion. A brief overview of the participants is presented in Table 5.1. The personal opinions expressed by the participants in the FGDs do not necessarily reflect the views of their organisation.

**Table 5.1**  Participants of the focus groups

| FG1 | Name | Information |
|---|---|---|
| | **Charisse (Chang) Jordan** | Programme Officer of the Safe and Fair Programme with UN Women Philippines |
| | **Emma Rhule** | Senior Researcher the United Nations University—International Institute for Global Health; Secretariat, Lancet Commission on Gender and Global Health |
| | **Jonathan Cohen** | Director of Policy Engagement at the USC Institute on Inequalities in Global Health |
| | **Marie Meudec** | Senior Social Scientist in the Outbreak Research Team // Population Data Hub, Equity & Health Unit, Department of Public Health, Institute of Tropical Medicine, Belgium |
| | **Salma El-Gamal** | Public Health Specialist |
| | **Sandhya Kanaka Yatirajula** | Senior Research Fellow at The George Institute for Global Health in New Delhi |
| **FG2** | | |
| | **Oriana López Uribe** | Member of Vecinas Feministas and RESURJ |
| | **Shehnaz Munshi** | Member of the Steering Committee of the People's Health Movement; Honourary Lecturer, School of Public Health, University of the Witwatersrand |
| | **Shubha Chacko** | Executive Director of the Indian NGO Solidarity Foundation |
| **FG3** | | |
| | **Awa Naghipour** | Co-founder of Feministische Medizin e.V; Medical researcher at the Department of Sex and Gender Sensitive Medicine, Medical Facutly OWL, Bielefeld University |
| | **Deborah Leticia Akumu** | Advocacy and Networking Officer at the Ugandan NGO OGERA |

A third participant representing a feminist organisation in Eastern Europe was unable to attend at short notice.

## 5.4      Data Collection and Analysis

This chapter presents how the online focus groups were conducted to collect the
required data for analysis, the process of transcription, and the qualitative content
analysis according to Kuckartz.

### 5.4.1   Data Collection Process and Transcription

After the participants confirmed their participation, a convenient date for everyone involved was jointly sought with the tool Doodle. FG1 was scheduled for
23 August 2022 at 13:00 CET. FG2 two took place on 24 August 2022 at
16:00 CET, and FG3 on 7 September 2022 at 18:00 CET. Prior to the sessions,
a comprehensive concept note was sent to all participants, including information on housekeeping, background, procedure, and participants regarding the
focus groups. Information about ethical considerations can be obtained from
Section 5.7.
    The focus groups were conducted with the audio-visual tool Zoom. The ses-
sions were audio and video recorded. FG1 lasted 120 minutes, FG2 106 minutes,
and FG3 98 minutes. All groups started with an introduction by the moderator (researcher), including housekeeping rules and background of the research
project. The discussion was initiated with a question addressed to everyone. Guiding questions were developed in advance, yet provided flexibility to ensure an
open discussion. They were categorised as *Challenges in global health*, *Alternatives and components of FGHP*, *Actors and accountability*, and *Action and
implementation*. The background of participants was considered by focusing
slightly more on the global scope in FG1, and rather on the local scope in FG2
and FG3. However, this was subject to the free flow of the discussion. Consistent
with feminist principles and as required for focus groups, the moderator remained
rather in the background. Interaction between the participants was encouraged as
well as the opportunity to include new aspects.

*Transcription*
On the basis of the audio-video recordings, the focus groups were transcribed,
i.e. converted into written language. As recommended by Kuckartz (2016) and
Dresing and Pehl (2018), a literal transcription was employed, neither phonetic nor
summarised. Approximation to written English, regarding language and punctu-
ation, was intended. Sentence form and language usage of the participants were
retained, including filler words. This indicates a compromise between an accurate

and comprehensible transcription (Kuckartz, 2016). A content-semantic transcript was generated with the purpose of focusing on content as well as interaction. Consistent with the objective of the research, more than the spoken word was transcribed, in particular approving or disapproving interactions. In adaption to the transcription notation by Dresing and Pehl (2018), the following rules were applied (Table 5.2):

**Table 5.2**  Transcription notation based on Dresing & Pehl (2018)

| (…) | Break up to 3 seconds |
| --- | --- |
| **(number)** | Break longer than 3 seconds, duration in brackets |
| <u>**underlined**</u> | Particular emphasis |
| **(nonverbal)** | Nonverbal expression |
| **(unint.)** | Unintelligible speech |
| **(word?)** | Unintelligible, assumed speech |
| **ehm** | Uniform notation of filler words (ehm, ah, eh) |
| / | Interruption of word or sentence |
| // | Speech overlaps |

Each contribution is presented as a separate paragraph, identified by assignable initials and the respective timestamp. In addition to the transcript, a memo was prepared by the researcher after each focus group, including thoughts, notes, and feelings about the content and atmosphere of the discussions (Dresing & Pehl, 2018; Kuckartz, 2016).

## 5.4.2  Qualitative Content Analysis

The analysis was conducted according to Kuckartz' (2016) qualitative content analysis due to its suitability for focus groups. Qualitative content analysis is a systematic approach based on the formulation of codes. With Kuckartz' (2019) words, codes lie "at the heart of the method" (p. 182) and are therefore essential for a qualitative content analysis. The data analysis process is described subsequently and visualised in Figure 5.1.

**Fig. 5.1** Data analysis
process

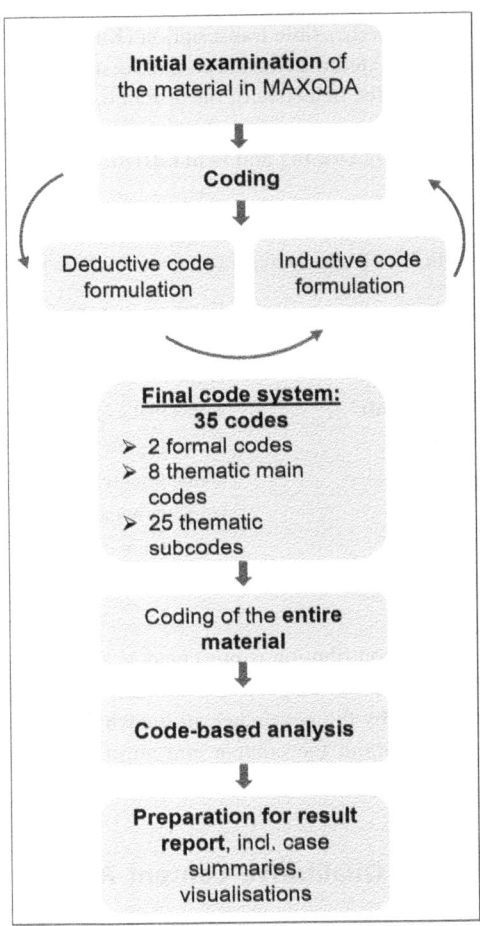

The transcripts and memos were inserted into the QDA-software MAXQDA for analysis. In an initial stage, the text material was examined through a hermeneutic approach (Kuckartz, 2016). In a second step, the material was coded. A deductive-inductive code formulation was employed, as suggested by Kuckartz (2016). At first, deductive codes were created on the basis of the guiding questions, i.e. *Challenges, Components of FGHP, Actors of FGHP,* and *Actions for*

*FGHP.* Subsequently, inductive main codes evolving from the material were identified, followed by subcodes. In a first round, all three transcripts were analysed with the deductive and inductive codes. The codes applied were predominantly thematic codes, encompassing specific topics, and two formal codes. Throughout the analysis it became apparent that the deductive codes had to be adjusted and new inductive main and subcodes were included. This happened in an iterative process. When the main and subcodes were regarded as final, the entire material was coded once more with the differentiated code system. The final code system entails ten main codes and 25 subcodes. Figure 5.2 portrays the thematic main and subcodes (without formal codes *Nonverbal & Interaction* and *Information about Participants*).

For a clear understanding and differentiation of the codes, they have been defined and summarised. Due to the complexity of the topic, frequent overlaps between codes occur. However, each code can be justified because different foci are identified. Explanations for the codes were depicted in a code system, including interlinkages with and differentiations from similar codes. Moreover, these

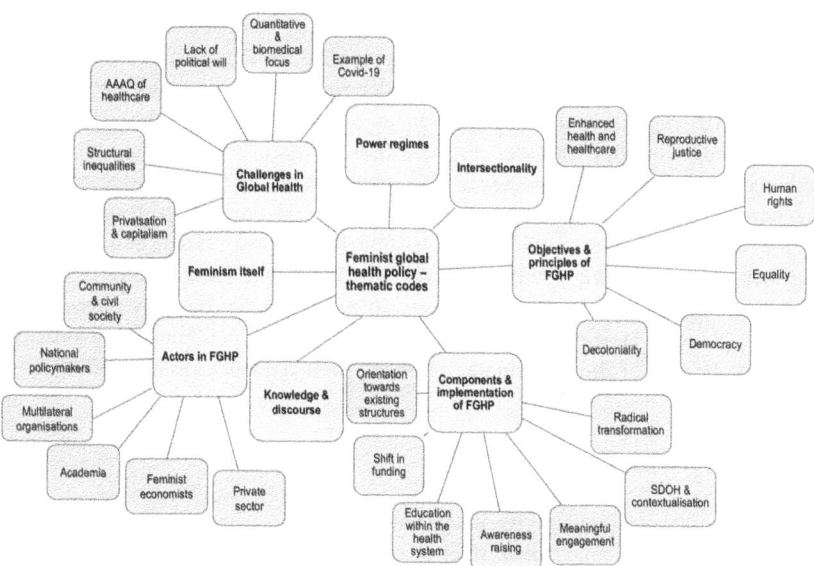

**Fig. 5.2** Visualisation of the code system with thematic main and sub codes

linkages emphasise the need for an intersectional understanding and the importance of structural approaches. A comprehensive hierarchical code system, which entails name, definition, scope of application and demarcation to other codes, and an anchor quote, was developed. The code-based analysis serves to answer the research question "How can a feminist approach to global health policy be meaningfully implemented to reduce health inequalities?" as the codes provide information to establish a framework for a FGHP and identify recommendations for a meaningful implementation. The qualitative content analysis was conducted based on the content of the codes, including information about interaction, and the interrelationships between the codes. For each focus group a case summary was prepared with respect to the research question, as described by Kuckartz (2016). Furthermore, a sensible sequence for the presentation of the results was developed as well as supportive visualisations.

## 5.5    Member Reflection

In alignment with feminist principles, a first draft of the results was sent to the participants, who were encouraged to provide feedback and requests for changes. Because the results are highly contextual, this approach was intended to ensure that participants felt correctly understood and agreed with the findings. Tracy (2010) regards member reflection as an instrument to enhance credibility by "providing opportunities for questions, critique, feedback, affirmation, and even collaboration." (p. 844). This participatory element shifts power to the participants. It allows for more meaningful and practicable results, which do not solely serve the researcher. Consistent with a postmodern understanding, member reflection acknowledges positionality. In this regard, Olmos-Vega and colleagues (2022) consider it as one way to practice reflexivity, as presented in the next chapter. However, reviewing the results is a time-demanding process. Accordingly, two of the participants provided their feedback on the findings.

## 5.6    Reflexivity

The incorporation of reflexivity is critical for post-positivist research and feminist methods in particular. Since science is not considered neutral and value-free, subjectivity and positionality of the researcher and participants highly impact the research process and outcomes (Wilkinson, 1988). Consistent with postmodernism, the socially constructed reality of the researcher and its influence should be acknowledged, not least to identify persisting power regimes in the research process. Reflexivity is furthermore important when conducting qualitative health research (Olmos-Vega et al., 2022). Olmos-Vega and colleagues (2022) highlight that while recognition of subjectivity is important, it is not sufficient if it does not result in appropriate action. They define reflexivity as

> a set of continuous, collaborative, and multifaceted practices through which researchers self-consciously critique, appraise, and evaluate how their subjectivity and context influence the research processes. (Olmos-Vega et al., 2022, p. 2)

In this regard, reflexivity should be considered throughout the whole research process. In their practical guide Olmos-Vega and colleagues (2022) identified mechanisms to include reflexivity, including reflexive writing by the researcher. In addition to individual reflexivity, the interpersonal relation between participants and researcher should be considered. For research teams, collaborative reflexivity is likewise important. This also entails member reflection, presented in Section 5.5, as it provides space for the participants to reflect on the results and suggest adjustments (Olmos-Vega et al., 2022).

Accordingly, my positionality will be presented briefly, including my background, experience, expectation, and motivation concerning this research. The first person singular is used intentionally to underline the subjectivity—and its importance. I am a 26 years old, white woman from Germany, a Global North country. I hold a bachelor's degree in Health Communication and I am enrolled in the master programmes Public Health and Political Science at the University of Bielefeld. This research is conducted as part of my master's thesis. My interest in the research topic is strongly motivated by personal experiences. I identify as female, my pronouns being she/her, and I am also perceived as female by society. I consider myself a feminist. I have previously worked with several non-governmental organisations in the field of global health policy and human rights in the German context. While I have a genuine interest to encounter the disciplines of public/global health and political science from a feminist perspective, my practical knowledge of feminist research is limited to my master programmes. I feel a strong urge to challenge social injustices, but I am simultaneously aware of my highly privileged position as a white, middle-class, German woman, who enjoys higher education. I was unknown to the participants previous to the focus groups. I consider them more experienced than me, regarding their lived experience as well as academic, research or work experience. By applying feminist research methods, I intend to dismantle power asymmetries within the research and to avoid exploitation. However, I am aware that power hierarchies remain due to my positionality. Firstly, because I am a white woman from a Global North country. The mere fact that I am able to conduct this research is a great privilege. Furthermore, I decided who was included in the focus groups. Secondly, the results of this research serve primarily to acquire my master's degree, even if the participants decide to use the results for their own purposes. Consequently, this research is strongly influenced by my positionality. In accordance with postmodernism, the analysis and findings are subjective and contextualised. Therefore, a researcher with a different positionality would have obtained deviating results.

## 5.7    Ethical Approval

Consistent with ethical principles for research, ethical approval for this study was obtained from the Ethics Committee of Bielefeld University (Nr. 2022–169). All participants were informed in advance about procedure, content, purpose, their rights, use of data, and data security. To this regard, two documents in accordance with the regulations of the University of Bielefeld were sent to them, namely the *Participation information and informed consent* and *Data protection declaration*. As this research is based on feminist research methods, anonymisation of participants was not intended to avoid objectification and exploitation. The objective of feminist research is to create more visibility and awareness and give voice to marginalised people, hence anonymisation would have been counter intuitive. The focus groups were audio and video recorded as emphasis is on the interaction between the participants in addition to what is being said. In accordance with this approach, all participants were invited to use the results and recordings for their own purposes. Use by third parties was not allowed. Written informed consent was obtained by all participants prior to the focus groups.

# Framework for a Feminist Global Health Policy

In this chapter the results identified through the focus groups to answer the research question "How can a feminist approach to global health policy be meaningfully implemented to reduce health inequalities?" are presented. Based on the qualitative content analysis according to Kuckartz (2016), a framework for a feminist global health policy is generated, including references for implementation. The components derived from the code-based analysis are depicted subsequently. The results are presented in aggregated form for each code with reference to the respective focus group or participant. Figure 6.1 portrays the thematic main and subcodes and provides an overview of the coding for each focus group (without the formal codes "Nonverbal & Interaction" and "Information about Participants"). However, this matrix is based on frequencies and should be interpreted with caution, as coded passages can be of different length, and quantity does not equal quality.

The focus groups further demonstrated the complexity of this topic. As presented in Figure 6.2, the thematic codes are highly interlinked, emphasising the relevance of a structural, holistic approach. In addition to what is being said, context and interaction of focus groups are important to consider. A vibrant discussion emerged in all three groups. In general, participants had a lot to contribute, and the discussions involved everyone. Interaction occurred mainly in the form of agreement, to reinforce statements by nodding and smiling.[1] Participants integrated further aspects that were not covered by the moderator, as anticipated when conducting focus groups. The duration of the focus groups depended on the group size. FG1, which consisted of the most participants, allowed the richest interaction. Concurrently, the smaller group size in FG2 and FG3 resulted in a higher proportion of speech for each participant. The atmosphere in all focus

---

[1] Agreement with statements is indicated in the analysis with+A after the initials.

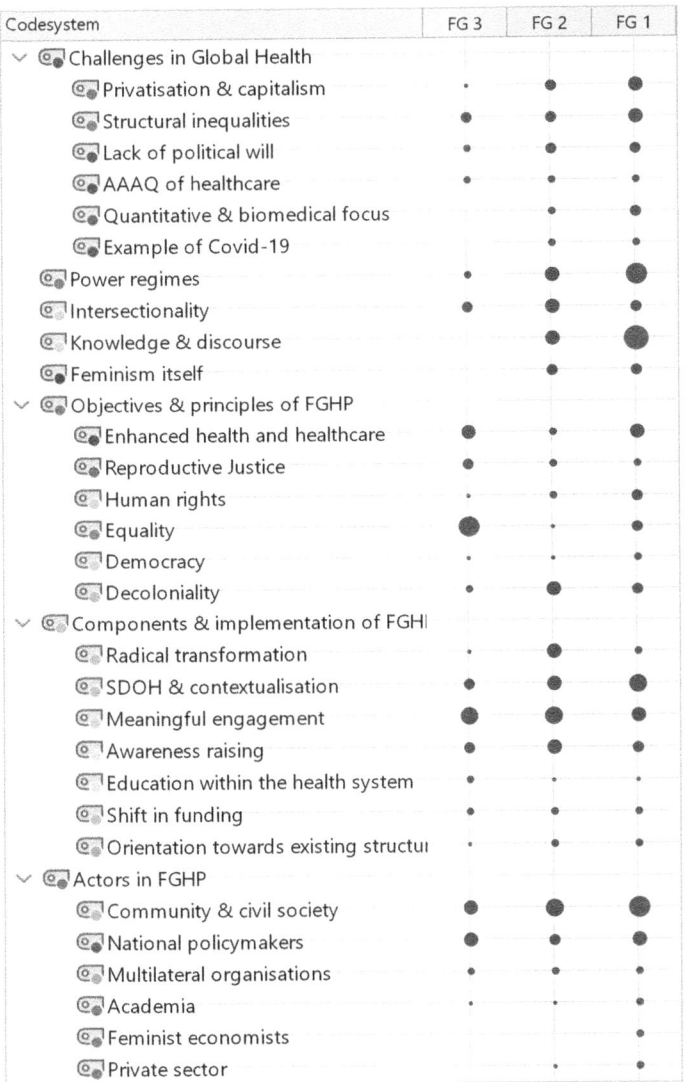

**Fig. 6.1** Code-Matrix-Browser of thematic codes. (Created with MAXQDA)

groups was very pleasant and congenial. In FG2 it was the most informal. All participants expressed to have enjoyed the exchange.

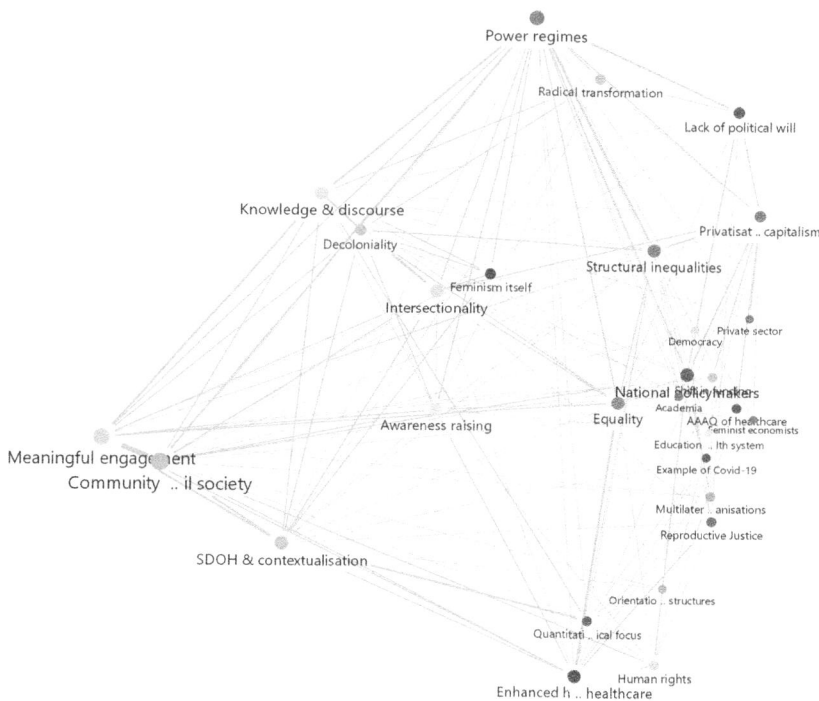

**Fig. 6.2**   Visualisation of the interlinkages of the codes. (Created with MAXQDA)

## 6.1   Challenges in Global Health

A comprehensive understanding of challenges is crucial to develop adequate alternatives—an often disregarded step, according to Marie (FG1, MM+A, 612–15). Major current structural challenges in global health were depicted by all participants. A high level of agreement was reached within and between the focus groups. Because of their structural character, the challenges are closely interrelated and interdependent, yet each represents a specific problem to be addressed.

### Privatisation & capitalism

Mentioned as one of the main challenges in all focus groups, particularly emphasised in FG1 and FG2, are the consequences of capitalism and privatisation on healthcare.

Capitalism more generally was regarded as ubiquitous in everyone's lives (FG2, OLU, 891–94). Participants of FG1 and FG2 mentioned how it enhances other power hierarchies, consistent with an intersectional understanding (e.g. FG1, CJ+A, 186–90). Regarding the health system, capitalistic and neoliberal structures serve to exploit healthcare workers. Given that the health workforce is highly gendered, this predominantly affects women (FG1, MM, 664–68; FG1, JC, 682–88; FG2, SC+A, 470–75). Emma further stated that these power hierarchies severely influence multilateral organisations in global health in the form of "philanthro-capitalists" (FG1, ER, 330).

More specifically, all participants agreed on privatisation in the health system as deeply concerning (e.g. FG1, SKY+A, 250–73; FG2, SC+A, 173–87; FG3, LDA, 524–34). Privatisation, resulting from capitalism, intersects with further oppressing power regimes, which increases inequalities (e.g. FG2, OLU, 555–56). The private sector turned far too influential in global health, nationally (e.g. FG2, SC, 173–87) as well as globally (e.g. FG1, ER, 322–33). Capitalistic profit-orientation, in contrast to prioritising health, is a threat leading to deleterious health impacts (e.g. FG1, SKY, 250–73; FG2, OLU, 556–57). This aspect was exemplified by Jonathan who referred to various "kinds of unregulated industries" (FG1, JC, 226) that endanger people's health. Unlike governments, the private sector is not accountable to society. Funding mechanisms do not need to be based on human rights or transparent principles (e.g. FG1, JC + A, 222–25; FG2, SC + A, 182–87). This endangers affordability and equal access to healthcare (FG2, SC + A, 178–82). Due to a lack of political will, the private sector remains unregulated (e.g. FG1, SKY, 264–72; FG3, LDA, 524–34). Not seldom because individual policymakers—more so in non-democratic states—may benefit from this system (FG1, JC, 235–49).

Given the inherent power dimension, this code is strongly linked to the codes "Power regime" and "Intersectionality". The problems depicted also entail suggestions for anticipated "Actors in FGHP" and questions around accountability. Furthermore, this code is closely related to the other identified challenges in the focus groups, which will be portrayed in detail subsequently.

## Structural inequalities

Structural inequalities are perceived as cross-cutting challenge and mentioned in all focus groups. They are related to the other subcodes and constitute either the cause or consequence of problems in global health. Inequalities arise from power hierarchies that rely on controlling, dehumanising, and feeling superior towards perceived others (e.g. FG1, CJ + A, 465–473; FG2, SM, 346–51). Structural inequalities are a global phenomenon, particularly apparent in coloniality and global classism. Examples in the focus groups included devaluing different medical knowledge (FG2, SC, 273–78) and exclusionary visa policies (FG3, LDA, 675–79). Structural power inequalities are deeply embedded within global health (FG1, ER, 292–304; FG1, MM, 392–95; FG2, SM, 387–95) and hence determine who is being heard and listened to (FG1, ER + A, 794–804; FG2, OLU, 420–428). The participants emphasised "the intersection of ehm structural inequalities" (FG1, CJ, 182), mainly referring to patriarchy, sexism and gender inequality, but also capitalism, colonialism, and racism (e.g. FG1, CJ + A, 189–90; FG2, OLU 445–57). Structural inequalities negatively affect health outcomes by restricting access to healthcare or leading to differential treatment based on discrimination (FG1, SKY, 276–83; FG2, SC + A, 232–47; FG3, AN, 768–72). The relevance of the political level was stressed to address these inequalities. However, Salma stated that policies frequently neglect "people that fall in between the cracks, people from intersectional groups" (FG1, SE + A, 354–55). Structural inequalities are inherently linked to power regimes and require an intersectional perspective to be genuinely addressed. A holistic approach to get to the root of the problems was regarded as essential to eliminate structural inequalities and hence improve health (e.g. FG1, CJ, 628–37; FG2, OLU, 800–07; FG3, LDA, 288–92).

## AAAQ of healthcare

Availability, accessibility, acceptability, and quality (AAAQ) of healthcare was a prominent topic in the discussions, as the overall objective was related to reduce health inequalities and improve health. This subcode indicates that multiple problems must be addressed.

Participants mentioned that UHC, which should entail AAAQ, has not been achieved so far (FG3, LDA, 190–99). Oriana further criticised the financial and quantitative orientation of this approach and demanded a focus on universal health care and true access instead of coverage, indicating that the quality of services is important as well (FG2, OLU, 188–96). Nonetheless, financial aspects, in particular the payment and high cost of services, were regarded as major issue regarding accessibility and affordability of healthcare. This is closely linked to privatisation and its restriction on access and equality, mainly prompted by profit-orientation and lack of accountability (FG1, JC, 225–35; FG3, LDA, 712–16). Shubha outlined the consequences, emphasising that privatisation

> has implications for access, it has implications for affordability (Oriana nods), it has implications about what kind of treatments get pushed, and what get ehm left out or neglected. Ehm, it has implications for ehm, who gets it, who will get access (Oriana nods), you know, which which class of people, which location of people, which kinds of people. (FG2, SC, 178–82)

Unmet AAAQ is an intersectional challenge as multiple power regimes constitute a barrier, affecting marginalised people the worst (FG1, SKY + A, 250–65; FG1, SE + A, 349–55). In FG2, the gendered inequality was emphasised, with Shubha and Oriana depicting that especially women are affected by limited access to healthcare. This is rooted in societal perceptions that determine gender inequality and thus unequal health (FG2, OLU, 211–18; FG2, SC, 232–47).

### *Lack of political will*
The "lack of (…) political will" (FG2, OLU, 500) to change the system as well as the preference for the status quo was a recurring topic in all focus groups. It was frequently mentioned that people in power are unwilling to give it up and thus blocking required progress and change. For instance, Awa stated that "those in power obviously ehm want to cling to it" (FG3, AN, 513), Sandhya explained "one of the reasons why they don't adopt feminist approaches is because it would then upset the apple cart" (FG1, SKY, 531–32), and Shehnaz shared:

> I don't know if those in power are willing to share their power (Oriana nods). The fact that people hold onto their power is dangerous. If powerful actors were not afraid to give away, distribute and share their power, we would have a more equitable world. I think that we have to start facing how much we love power (…) we are not satisfied (…) we always want more power. (FG2, SM, 823–28)

Questioning the status quo and intending change would imply a radical transformation, which was considered undesirable by policymakers (e.g. FG2, OLU, 515–27). The reason for this reluctance lies in personal convenience, as noted by Charisse "they continue the status quo because they benefit from it" (FG1, CJ, 633–34) and elaborated by Sandhya:

> to address that would mean, then, that you have to have a more equitable distribution of resources (Emma and Marie nod) and really question fundamental things which are

easier left as they are (Emma and Jonathan nod) because then you're able to continue exercising the power (FG1, SKY, 536–39)

This partly explains the lack of regulation and monitoring of the private sector, which poses a major obstacle to health equality (FG1, JC, 235–49). From an intersectional perspective, people in power only serve specific interests, mostly in favour of the dominant power regime (FG2, OLU, 554–59). Hence, there exists no interest for those dominating to include the community and shift power (FG1, MM, 367–74).

### Quantitative & biomedical focus

Participants of FG1 and FG2 referred to the narrow biomedical and quantitative focus in global health as concerning. Global health and medicine are regarded from a predominantly biomedical lens, neglecting the social determinants of health and the context (FG1, ER + A, 406–415, FG1, JC + A, 485–515). This causes negative health impacts. Orientation towards treatment and cure disregards prevention and the need to address the causes of problems. Accordingly, underlying power dynamics and inequalities that influence health are not considered—impeding a more sustainable approach (FG1, ER, 409–15; FG2, SC + A, 531–44). The participants reported a strong resistance within global health on more holistic approaches that take the SDOH, intersectionality, and qualitative indicators into consideration (FG1, ER + A, 402–29). The biomedical frame is taught in the medical education, reproducing its dominance (FG1, SKY + A, 273–91). According to the participants, the preference for quantitative indicators is visible across global health, in policymaking as well as research. While being regarded as measurable and comparable, these indicators often fail to reflect reality—not least because they are neglecting the context and circumstances. As Marie stated, "there is no focus on the impactful change, there's no focus on the process and only on the output." (FG1, MM, 382–83). Jonathan introduced the term "biomedical solutionism" (FG1, JC, 486) to describe this phenomenon. Policymakers prefer to present convenient results—irrespective of their relevance. Consistently, the quantification of the SDGs was mentioned as one of their major shortcomings (FG1, SKY + A, 334–47; FG2, OLU, 642–54). A quantitative and biomedical approach further emphasises coloniality within global health. By defining what counts as facts, other knowledge systems are devalued and regarded as unscientific (FG1, ER, 398–426; FG2, SC, 253–62). The quantitative orientation is influenced by privatisation and capitalism, as these systems rely on financial aspects and demand numerical data to measure progress.

This affects global health research and universities, which are adapting to these external pressures (FG1, MM + A, 380–83).

To demonstrate the shortcomings of a quantitative and biomedical frame, the Covid-19 pandemic was used as an example by the participants. Since it presents a significant current global health crisis and was mentioned by participants in FG1 and FG2 several times, the example of Covid-19 is a subcode on its own.

***Example of Covid-19***
Examples of the Covid-19 pandemic were given to portray persisting inequalities that became visible and were reinforced through the pandemic. Participants of FG1 and FG2 presented that pandemic responses—particularly in the beginning—were too narrow, relying on a biomedical and quantitative scope. The context and SDOH were not taken into account (FG1, CJ, 204–11; FG1, JC, 496–504). The participants agreed that a comprehensive approach would have significantly improved health outcomes and saved lives, as health inequalities mainly arose from structural causes (FG1, ER + A, 404–12; FG1, JC, 496–504). The example of Covid-19 demonstrates the dysfunctionality of the current system, which disproportionately affects the most marginalised, especially in times of crisis. Hence, the necessity of a new system and transformation is emphasised (FG2, OLU, 798–807).

## 6.2    Power Regimes

Power regimes were a central theme throughout all focus groups. Reference to power were made with regard to the negative side, i.e. problematic power hierarchies, unequal distribution of power and its consequences, as well as from a forward-looking perspective, i.e. how existing power regimes can be changed and create more equality. The role of power is of high importance for analysing existing problems and generating feminist alternatives. Due to this outstanding relevance, the code "Power regime" is an independent code. It is a cross-cutting topic and therefore reappears in almost every other code.

Power asymmetries and their adverse impact were alluded by all participants. Power regimes are persistent globally. Unequal structures cause oppression and domination (FG1, CJ, 183–86; FG2, SM + A, 343–64). Participants of FG1 and FG2 elaborated that power is related to whose interests are being served, who is included and able to speak (FG1, MM + A,367–80; FG2, SM + A, 397–407; FG3, AN, 229–38). Consistent with an intersectional understanding, different power regimes and their interlinkages were addressed. Examples mainly related to patriarchy, racism and colonialism, and classism and capitalism (e.g. FG1, SKY, 277–291; FG2, SM + A, 366–71; FG3, AN, 506–10). These intersecting power dimensions negatively affect health. Charisse referred to the risks for SRHR due to "the interplay amongst patriarchy, sexism, heteronormativity, and ehm, the role of ehm ehm the capitalist and ehm you know, ehm neoliberal structures" (FG1, CJ, 188–90). As stated in the subcode "Lack of political will", power regimes are tenacious. The persistence of power hierarchies demands radical change because only by transforming structures progress can be achieved (e.g. FG1, SKY, 531–42; FG2, SM + A, 397–407).

The global health system itself is likewise infiltrated by power hierarchies, as Emma noted "power inequities are really baked into the global health architecture" (FG1, ER, 293–94). Examples of power hierarchies at institutional level were presented from the medical system (FG1, SKY, 277–91), academia (FG2, OLU, 449–457), and feminist movements (FG3, AN, 517–20). Unequal power dynamics are reproduced at individual level (FG3, LDA, 286–92). However, above all, the power of the private sector in global health was highlighted—with Oriana's words, "They have more power than most of the/ our government." (FG2, OLU, 664–65).

The participants also indicated the role of power for feminist global health policy and the required change. Charisse summarised that

> "It's also about how can we dismantle this ehm this ehm this structure, this dominant structure that perpetuates inequality, and perpetuates ehm very oppressive, discriminating, ehm and repressive health policies." (FG1, CJ, 635–37)

Awa mentioned the necessity to raise awareness and "involving everyone" (FG3, AN, 229). The inclusion and participation of the community and a bottom-up approach was regarded as essential in all focus groups to advance a shift in power (e.g. FG1, SE + A, 709–19; FG2, SM, 713–17; FG3, AN, 489–97). The aspect of power is crucial when considering the components for a FGHP, which are presented in detail in Sections 6.6 and 6.7.

The participants, especially in FG1, also introduced meta-level discourses about power. They considered the characteristics of power, whether it can be shared and is indefinite or whether a shift in power is associated with a loss of it. FG1 rather agreed on a "mutualising view of power" (FG1, JC, 595) and the assumption that a shift is beneficial for everyone, rejecting the zero-sum idea based on a "commodification of power" (FG1, JC, 596). However, this remains an open discussion as it was also indicated that some people might have to give up power (e.g. FG1, ER + A, 561–86; MM + A, 601–09).

## 6.3    Intersectionality

Intersectionality, as well as power, is an overarching theme that relates to both, the challenges and the way forward. It is inherently linked to power regimes, as per definition intersectionality refers to multiple interconnected power dynamics. Accordingly, aspects related to intersectionality reappear in various codes. Regarding the significance of an intersectional approach, its analysis requires a separate code.

The relevance of intersectionality as comprehensive frame to ensure a holistic approach to a FGHP was frequently emphasised in all discussions (e.g. FG1, JC, 962–63; FG3, LDA, 248–53). FG3 highlighted that an intersectional perspective is pivotal to involve everyone in the policy-making process (FG3, AN, 228–35). This approach is further relevant to achieve UHC and health equality (FG2, SM, 707–11; FG3, LDA, 190–92). According to the participants, intersectionality enables the recognition of different needs and how to adequately respond to these (FG3, LDA, 401–07). Consistently, feminism itself must be inherently intersectional (e.g. FG1, MM + A, 741–55; FG2 SM + A, 374–79). To develop alternatives, awareness about pervasive intersecting discriminations is indispensable (FG2, SM + A, 366–73; FG3, LDA, 262–73).

## 6.4    Knowledge & Discourse

Considerations about knowledge and discourse were predominantly shaped by FG1 and FG2. They included meta-level questions regarding knowledge paradigms as well as more direct approaches to knowledge, discourse, and language. A rather abstract discussion highlighted the need to consider and rethink fundamental assumptions.

Participants emphasised the importance to recognise that knowledge paradigms are not neutral but rather shaped by power (FG1, CJ, 473–75; FG2, SC, 494–99). This includes what accounts for knowledge as well as the use of language. Accordingly, a "sense of imagination" (FG2, SM, 685) and a "shift in mindset" (FG1, JC, 832) are required to think outside the common frames. Further reflections referred to the definitions of global health and power (FG1, ER, 302–12; 561–86; FG2, OLU, 300–06, 420, SM, 840–42). Less abstractly, discourse and power were discussed with regard to who is part of the conversation and listened to (FG1, CJ + A, 209–11, 807–31; MM + A, 370–72). Related to these considerations, a turn to community and "lived experience"

(FG1, ER, 415) was demanded (FG1, MM, 378–79; FG2, SM, 718–27). Reflections on knowledge and discourse are closely associated with colonialism. Firstly, because existing knowledge paradigms are influenced by a Western perspective, which often devalues other knowledge system, and secondly because coloniality determines who shapes the discourse (FG1, ER, 421–24; FG2, SM + A, 383–90). Shehnaz highlighted the continuing influence of colonialism by stating that "even the very fact that we're having this conversation in English, yet we are from three different continents" (FG2, SM, 687–88). These fundamental assumptions are important to consider with regard to FGHP. This code is therefore relevant to all codes and their outcomes.

## 6.5   Feminism Itself

When dealing with a feminist approach to policy, it is critical to engage with feminism itself first. This was mentioned a few times in FG1 and FG2. As Emma highlighted, "feminism does not equal women" (FG1, ER, 780), but is rather a holistic and intersectional approach. The participants further agreed on the existence of plural feminisms in contrast to one singular approach (FG1, MM + A, 741–47; ER + A, 766–71). In this regard, feminisms must be intersectional and contextualised (FG1, MM + A, 748–55; ER, 977–1004). The colonial and racist history of the feminist movement, which was shaped by mainly white, middle-class educated women, was an important concern in the discussions (FG1, FG2, SM + A, 374–84). Shehnaz emphasised that "we can't go into feminist policy if we're not taking history seriously. We need to understand histories of oppression and of feminist resistance" (FG2, SM, 383–84). The impact is still visible today, as the movement itself struggles with power hierarchies, including exclusionary mechanisms (FG1, JC + A, 954–76; FG2, OLU, 786–93). Hence, internal improvements are required. Not least due to the threat of anti-feminist movements (FG1, ER, 942–53), feminism should be appealing to the broader population. Participants suggested reflecting on power asymmetries, aligning words with action, and improving communication (FG1; JC + A, 955–57; FG2, OLU; 909–19, SM, 926–31).

## 6.6    Objectives & Principles of FGHP

The overall objectives of a feminist global health policy and the underlying fundamental principles, extracted from the focus groups, are presented below. Highlighted in the discussions, a focus on solutions is not appropriate, as this indicates single, easy-to-achieve mechanisms (FG1, JC + A, 488–94). Complex problems demand a "pluriversality of approaches" (FG1, ER, 767). Therefore, the term *alternatives* is applied instead of *solutions* for a feminist global health policy, to emphasise the complexity and multiplicity—of new approaches as well as challenges.

### Enhanced health and healthcare

One of the major objectives of a FGHP referred to by the participants was enhanced health and healthcare. The importance of this outcome was depicted in all focus groups, in particular in FG3. An improved healthcare provision leading to better health and quality of life is anticipated (e.g. FG3, LDA, 248–50). The participants discussed the necessary requirements to achieve this. A structural change, including power transformation, is indispensable (FG2, OLU, 795–98). To ensure "comprehensive and holistic health services" (FG2, LDA, 730–31), the recognition of the SDOH and the context is crucial (e.g. FG1, SKY, 341–47). As Jonathan phrased it:

> I could not agree more that feminism, takes us ehm from a narrow focus on biomedical solutionism to a broader focus on wellness and health as a complete state of psychological, physical, mental, spiritual well-being (Chang nods), and an emphasis on the social determinants of health. (FG1, JC, 485–88)

This entails a shift away from the limited scope portrayed in Section 6.1. Equally important is an "sensitisation process" (FG3, AN, 339) at every level. Participants highlighted that change cannot happen without the support and inclusion of communities (e.g. FG1, ER + A, 421–29; FG2, SC + A, 229–32). For a health system to function, the (gendered) health workforce needs to be adequately valued, also in financial terms (FG2, SC, 460–81). Recognising intersectionality and diversity, universal access must be ensured while simultaneously acknowledging the needs of individuals (e.g. FG3, LDA, 401–07). Section 6.7 provides more detailed information about the components of a FGHP and how to reach the objectives.

The participants further indicated that enhanced health implies equality and an improvement of legal and political rights, thus emphasising health equality (FG3,

LDA, 309–14). More specifically, UHC is to be achieved as well as the fulfilment of SRHR and bodily autonomy (FG2, OLU, 328–32; FG3, LDA, 719–31). This aspect will be highlighted in the next section.

***Reproductive Justice***
The achievement of reproductive justice was emphasised as a second crucial objective. Closely related to health equality, this concept further encompasses social justice. Due to its relevance in feminist discourses, reproductive justice was frequently mentioned in the focus groups. Not least because it specifically demonstrates the importance of the political level and the relevance of power, here in the form of controlling (mainly) women's bodies (FG1, C + AJ, 179–90, 459–73). In the focus groups, SRHR was used as example, often focusing on the negative aspects, i.e. the colonial history of SRHR and the ongoing political and societal challenges preventing the fulfilment of SRHR (e.g. FG2, SM, 374–85; FG3, LDA, 293–99). Intersecting power hierarchies further exacerbate the situation for individuals and cause major inequalities (FG1, CJ + A, 186–90). However, hope was expressed that a FGHP has the potential to improve the situation. Laws and policies tremendously impact SRHR—sometimes with detrimental consequences. At the same time, they contain the opportunity to achieve reproductive justice (FG2, AN, 364–68). One aspect of reproductive justice mentioned by participants in all focus groups was "bodily autonomy and integrity" (FG3, LDA, 314) (FG1, JC, 528–30; FG2, OLU, 329–32; FG3, LDA, 320–28). Bodily autonomy implies a shift in power since more autonomy equals less hierarchy. Furthermore, it presents a necessity and goal for a FGHP and includes equality and rights—principles that are depicted subsequently.

***Human rights***
The fulfilment of human rights is central for a feminist global health policy. Participants from all focus groups highlighted the universal principles entailed in human rights as a required fundament for a FGHP (e.g. FG1, CJ, 853–55; FG3, LDA, 248–53). Human rights must be at the core of this approach, including the notion of health as a human right (FG1, CJ, 450–52; FG2, SC + A, 224–30).[2] Although contextualisation is of major importance—presented in Section 6.7— overarching principles that apply to everyone worldwide were regarded necessary (FG2, SC, 619–22, OLU, 645–47). Politics play an important role here. It is political responsibility to ensure human rights, especially considering the risk of rights

---

[2] The relevance of the Universal Declaration of Human Rights for a FGHP is presented in Section 6.7.

being restricted by privatisation in health (FG1, CJ, 441–46; SKY + A, 549–60; FG2, SC + A, 182–86). To ensure meaningful realisation of the human right to health, communities are essential. They facilitate education and consciousness-raising about human rights and empower people to live and act accordingly (FG1, SKY + A, 549–60; FG2, SC + A, 224–53). Deborah emphasised the role of "women human rights defenders" for the protection and promotion of human rights (FG3, LDA, 254). At the same time, it is crucial to ensure the rights of activists, as they are at risk when exposing injustices (e.g. FG3, LDA, 254–61). Human rights are closely aligned with the principle of equality, which is presented in the next section.

## *Equality*

Since a FGHP is inherently about health equality and focuses on gender equality, the principle of equality is essential. Particularly emphasised in FG3, it was discussed in all focus groups. Equality is closely related to social justice and human rights (FG1, JC + A, 222–25). It can only be achieved by acknowledging the underlying power hierarchies that cause inequalities. Since inequalities and power regimes are socially constructed, they can be challenged and changed through action (FG2, SM, 836–46; FG3, AN, 631–42). Consistent with an intersectional understanding, the participants highlighted that equality needs to be achieved through equity, i.e. acknowledging and acting according to everyone's (heterogenous) needs (FG1, ER + A, 773–79; FG3, LDA, 273–84, 401–07). Addressing equities first to achieve equality requires a shift in power. The overarching principle of equality is critical for a FGHP to be truly holistic. It was further noted that equality is key for UHC and reproductive justice (FG3, LDA, 309–14). As with all human rights, laws and policies are important for equality since they can either enhance or restrict equality (e.g. FG2, SM + A, 399–407). The participants emphasised that everyone must be included since equality can only be realised by meaningful participation (e.g. FG1, CJ + A, 828–31).

## *Democracy*

Human rights and equality indicate major components of democracy. The significance of this political system was mentioned, highlighted particularly in FG1 and more indirectly in FG2 and FG3 with reference to its basic principles. In addition to human rights and equality, democracy entails meaningful engagement and thus the distribution of power (e.g. FG3, AN, 342–47). Therefore, democracy is essential for a feminist global health policy. The (national) political context is decisive for adopting and implementing a FGHP (e.g. FG3, LDA, 535–39). Governments must be held accountable as they are responsible, which implies that participation of society at state level is critical (FG1, SE + A, 709–19; FG2, OLU, 571–84). Participants in FG1 emphasised the importance of democracy in contrast to authoritarianism, which poses a major threat not just for FGHP (FG1, JC, 240–49, SKY, 720–25). Jonathan further elaborated that non-democratic states are more prone to privatisation of healthcare, with major implications:

> I think that political leaders who ehm are not held to democratic checks and balances are much more likely to enter into sweetheart deals with corporations to be seduced by corporate lobbying to be bought, and so the erosion of democracy and the erosion of political checks and balances, and the balance of power between the executive branch, the legislative branch, the judicial branch is so profoundly linked to ehm the kind of corporate capture of healthcare because ultimately it's the decisions of political leaders in countries with weak governance and weak rule of law and rising authoritarianism ehm that permit corporate capture of public goods. So in some ways those two issues of authoritarianism and corporate capture are very linked. (FG1, JC, 240–49)

Authoritarianism is also linked to anti-feminist and anti-gender movements, not seldom combining sexist and racist assumptions (FG1, JC + A, 914–30). Accordingly, the political system of a state determines health and health outcomes of its population. This underlines the importance of democracy for a FGHP.

### *Decoloniality*
Since a feminist global health policy is inherently intersectional, decoloniality is one of its main principles. It was part of all discussions and strongly emphasised by Shehnaz in FG2. As a first step, "we have to acknowledge the history. We have to acknowledge the past." (FG2, SM, 341–42). Awareness about colonialism is critical, including reflection on intrinsic colonial assumptions (FG1, ER + A, 782–88; FG2, SM, 693–95). This is highly important to understand existing structures, i.e. who holds power, who is heard, whose interests are served (FG3, AN, 631–34). The impact of colonialism is still apparent today. This process of reflection is related to the considerations in Section 6.4 about knowledge and discourse, as knowledge paradigms are characterised by colonial premises (FG1, ER, 421–24; CJ + A, 807–11; FG2, SM, 384–88). The intersection of colonialism with other power regimes—particularly capitalism, patriarchy, and racism—determines resources, funding, and the distribution of power (FG2, SM + A, 340–73). Due to colonial and racist structures within feminist movements, an intersectional, anti-racist, and decolonial approach is essential (FG1, JC + A, 957–69; FG2, SM + A, 374–84). Decoloniality demands accountability from states of the Global North, bilaterally and within multilateral institutions (FG2, OLU, 655–61; FG3, AN, 631–42). Equality, equity, and social justice are key

components of a decolonial approach. Only by involving everyone it can be pursued (FG1, CJ, 807–13; FG3, LDA, 673–82). Individuals as well as institutions need to reflect on their positions and means of contribution (FG1, ER, 790–95; FG2, SM, 836–40). Advancing decoloniality is a complex challenge, demanding radical transformation (FG2, SM, 852–56). Due to this complexity, and as stated in the beginning of this chapter, there is no singular approach to decolonise, but rather multiple (FG1, ER, 768–72).

## 6.7    Components & Implementation of FGHP

As presented in the previous chapter, the participants agreed on universal principles for a FGHP, i.e. human rights, equality, democracy, and decoloniality. This chapter now focuses on how to comply with these principles to achieve health equality and reproductive justice. The code encompasses components of a FGHP and information about concrete implementation. Regarding the latter, emphasis is on local adaption, guided by universal principles. However, as with every global framework, it has to be flexible and adaptable. Shubha reinforced this aspect by highlighting:

> like with all feminist stuff, it has to be flexible and (more important?) it has to be work in progress […] it's going to be something that allows people to take what they want, add, eject, shape, reshape, you know. It has to be (...) ehm, you know, like clay or plastic, whatever, you know. Like clay where you can keep moulding and re-moulding it. (FG2, SC, 628–34)

Due to the complexity of such a framework, the subcodes presented subsequently are closely interlinked and should therefore not be considered in isolation.

### Radical transformation
The demand for a radical transformation to implement a FGHP was frequently endorsed in all focus groups, the most in FG2. The necessity of such radical change is rooted in the problem depicted in the subcode "Lack of political will". It became obvious that the current system is not functioning (e.g. FG2, OLU, 515–16, 667–69). The persistence of power regimes inherent in societies reproduces inequalities. Since some individuals, among them policymakers, are unwilling to change the status quo and share power, radical transformation of power systems is essential (e.g. FG2, SC, 492–96; FG2, OLU, 889–91). The participants elaborated

that such an approach requires "to think outside of the box" (FG2, OLU, 559–60) and adapt different perspectives (FG1, SKY, 541–43; FG2, SM, 738–41). Shehnaz further indicated that transforming a system demands time and is "going to be a very uncomfortable, difficult, hard process" (FG2, SM, 850). Shifting power further implies action on the ground. Awa as well as Shehnaz noted that society must get "angry" (FG2, SM, 858; FG3, AN, 758) of the current system to create space for change. Consistently, the term "revolution" (e.g. FG1, SKY, 542; FG2, SM, 853) was mentioned several times in the focus groups. Radical transformation paves the way for a FGHP that delivers critical improvements in health and equality (e.g. FG2, OLU, 328–29).

### SDOH & contextualisation

The relevance of acknowledging the social determinants of health and the context was strongly emphasised by all participants. Correspondingly, negligence of this aspect was perceived as one of the greatest challenges in global health (e.g. FG2, SC, 531–48). Frameworks in general should always consider local circumstances and context-specific adaption. The same accounts for a FGHP, which must be respectful of the contextual setting to be meaningful (e.g. FG1, MM, + A, 609–17; FG2, SM + A, 388–402; FG3, LDA, 607–13). Specified by Awa, "It needs to be ehm always thought in context of the local and resources, and whatever people need and ehm whatever place they are." (FG3, AN, 227–28). Moreover, Shubha elaborated that a FGHP

> has to be contextualised, and it has to be/ it has to make sense, you know, for you. But certain sort of broad principles, broad frameworks can be ehm developed, but it's important that those frameworks take into consideration (...) the local the, you know, and the state level, the regional level, at the international level, and and how these linkages can be established. (FG2, SC, 618–22)

Focusing on the context indicates recognition of the SDOH (FG1, JC + A, 485–88). As elaborated in Section 6.1, a biomedical and quantitative scope is insufficient to improve health outcomes and detrimental for bodily autonomy (FG1, JC + A, 526–30). Hence, more comprehensive approaches were deemed crucial by the participants (e.g. FG1, SKY + A, 338–47; FG2, OLU + A, 644–58). Contextualisation also entails the involvement of community because they are embedded in and aware of the context (e.g. FG1, MM, 374–80; FG2, SC, 474–83; FG3, LDA, 433–57). This aspect is further elaborated in the next section. Besides considering the SDOH and context of individuals to improve health, the structural context must be included as well—locally, nationally, and globally (FG1, ER +

A, 790–804; FG2, SC, 618–22). This entails the political context and power hierarchies. All participants highly emphasised that only by recognising the broader picture meaningful change can occur and advance health equality (e.g. FG1, SKY + A, 338–47; FG1, ER + A, 409–21).

### Meaningful engagement

The subcode "Meaningful engagement" is highly interrelated with the subcodes "SDOH & contextualisation" and "Community & civil society". While these codes closely align, each of them highlights particular aspects. The relevance of "Meaningful engagement" as an independent subcode is endorsed by being one of the most mentioned and elaborated topics in the discussions. It was referred to in all three focus groups exceedingly. Meaningful engagement constitutes a major component of a FGHP and entails information for purposeful implementation.

All participants agreed that a FGHP can only be successful by involving the community and civil society (e.g. FG3, LDA, 379–84). Enhanced health and healthcare require participatory approaches (FG1, ER + A, 421–29; FG2, OLU, 306–17, SC, 474–83). Only by involving people on the ground, the recognition of the SDOH and context is ensured (FG2, SC + A, 537–48; FG3, LDA, 446–67). This resonates with a decolonial approach, which cannot be pursued without meaningful engagement and acknowledging alternative kinds of knowledge (FG1, ER, 421–24; FG2, SM, 705–30). Participation is crucial for change regarding the political and legal level as well as the socio-cultural level. The participants of the focus groups indicated what meaningful engagement implies. The engagement of everyone—referring to the 2030 Agenda notion of leaving no one behind—was deemed significant (e.g. FG3, AN, 228–35, LDA, 673–82). The concept of intersectionality was highlighted in this respect, indicating that particularly marginalised and multiple oppressed individuals must be heard and not neglected (e.g. FG1, CJ + A, 828–31; FG2, OLU, 503–11; FG3, LDA, 262–73). Emphasising this approach, Awa stated that "we need to mirror society also in the policy-making processes" (FG3, AN, 231–32). Therefore, the engagement of local communities is integral, as they are knowledgeable about what works and is needed (FG2, SM, 718–37). In accordance, Shehnaz demanded that

we need to start listening differently. We need to stop turning to people who hold power and privilege for solutions. Those who don't have lived experiences of structural oppression don't understand the complex everyday reality navigating difficult conditions of poverty and inequality. So their solutions fall short. We've got to shift who we listen to. (FG2, SM, 712–19)

Consequently, community involvement constitutes the foundation of a FGHP (FG3, LDA, 379–84). Participants further pointed to the role of the political level. While emphasis was on the communities, the interlinkage of a bottom-up with a top-down approach was considered critical (FG2, SC, 474–83; FG3, AN, 368–74). It is political responsibility to ensure inclusion and participation—from the beginning. Participants emphasised that this must be done in an iterative, continuous process, which is time-consuming, but rewarding and essential (FG1, MM + A, 384–92; FG1, ER + A, 425–29; FG3, LDA, 433–35, AN, 661–65). Participatory approaches require change in institutions at every level (FG1, MM, 374–80). Awa and Deborah suggested to create adaptable mechanisms for engagement (FG3, LDA, 457–67, AN, 477–98). It was further highlighted in all focus groups that a FGHP must be understandable and relatable to the people (FG2, OLU, 907–19, SM, 962–64; FG3, AN, 220–24, LDA, 603–27).

Meaningful engagement is therefore a major component of a FGHP, linking various aspect. Listening to other voices and ensuring participation entails shifting power—a necessary prerequisite for making a FGHP inherently intersectional and decolonial. Furthermore, meaningful engagement is closely related to raising consciousness among all levels (FG2, SM, 863–67; FG3, AN, 631–42), which is further elaborated in the next section.

*Awareness raising*

Adopting a FGHP requires awareness raising. This component, encompassing several aspects, was mentioned in all focus groups. Participants referred to the necessity of being aware about who is in power, included, and heard. Understanding the status quo is critical for social change (FG2, OLU, 773–81; FG3, AN, 505–12). Raising awareness also relates to sensitising communities with regard to their rights and power hierarchies, to facilitate action based on that consciousness (FG1, SKY + A, 549–60; FG2, SC, 226–32; FG3, AN, 339–49, 756–66). Because, as Sandhya emphasised, meaningful change will only occur if "people realise that they have rights" (FG1, SKY, 550). Consequently, transforming the system demands awareness at every level. Once again, communities are vital to ensure this "sensitisation process" (FG3, AN, 339) as they are trusted and aware of the context (FG1, SKY + A, 657–61). Regarding the previously depicted aspect of meaningful engagement, policymakers likewise need to be aware of power hierarchies and ways to include the community (FG3, AN, 335–338, 368–71). The participants further discussed the relevance of acknowledging reflexivity and positionality. This refers to the awareness of one's own positionality and embeddedness in certain structures. It entails a reflection process about privileges and responsibility (FG1, ER + A, 317–20; FG2, SM, 743–47; FG3, AN,

631–42). These considerations are particularly important considering research, as positionality affects both the process and outcomes (FG3, AN, 413–17). Moreover, reflexivity concerns institutions as well as individuals (FG1, ER, 790–97; FG2, SM, 833–39). Developing a consciousness about the influence of one's position is thus essential for a FGHP.

### Education within the health system

This subcode is closely related to the previous subcode, "Awareness raising", since education is one way to advance awareness. However, this subcode has a slightly different focus, as it refers explicitly to the training and content taught to the health workforce and the respective education system. This aspect was mentioned a few times in all focus groups. The participants pointed to challenges concerning education in the health system. Harmful power asymmetries are persistent and continuously reproduced, including patriarchy, colonialism, racism, and classism (FG2, OLU, 449–57). Sandhya illustrated this problem for the Indian context:

> And another challenge that I would also like to touch upon is really the entire medical education and the way in which this education is given. So you know the principles of human rights, and all of that are not taught to medical practitioners (Jonathan and Salma nod). [...] So I feel the entire medical education has a lack of empathy. The lack of these skills, which you could call soft skills, are very, important, they're critical. But they're not part of the medical education. [...] If you come in with money, with power, with status, you would be guaranteed good treatment. Otherwise, ehm, it's your la/ luck basically whether you survive or not. (FG1, SKY, 273–90)

The criticised biomedical and quantitative scope is taught, thus preventing a more holistic approach with respect to the SDOH and contextualised knowledge. Consequently, improvements in health equality and health outcomes are compromised. Deborah also criticised the incomprehensible medical terminology that limits self-determination of patients (FG3, LDA, 624–27). A consciousness-expanding process among healthcare personnel is important to avoid the reproduction of power hierarchies within the health system (AN, 772–84). Ideally, this process is embedded in education and training of the health workforce from the beginning. This approach will not only improve the health of patients, but is further critical to advance decoloniality (FG3, AN, 758–63, 772–84).

*Shift in funding*
Regarding the challenges related to privatisation and capitalism portrayed in Section 6.1, a shift in funding was considered essential for a FGHP. Without adequate funding a framework cannot be meaningfully implemented (FG3, LDA, 524–34, AN, 637). Therefore, participants in all discussions demanded a change of funding mechanisms, "particularly given that money does equal power" (FG1, ER, 905–06). It was criticised that the current system is predominantly disadvantageous for the Global South and neglecting feminist approaches (FC1, JC, 683–90; FG3, LDA, 524–28). The participants depicted what a shift in funding should encompass. Instead of profits, health should be at the centre of funding decisions. The latter should also align to feminist principles (FG1, JC, 679–91; ER, 727–29, 897–906). Again, the engagement of communities—which are often underfunded—was considered crucial to achieve a meaningful impact (FG1, ER, 901–04; FG3, LDA, 528–34). A shift in funding implies transformation of power since it is decisive who has money (FG1, ER, 904–06; FG2, SM + A, 842–51). Oriana indicated that more action at state-level was required, proposing redistributive mechanisms, different taxation systems, and more allocation for healthcare and other social sectors (FG2, OLU, 317–22). Redistribution was also mentioned with reference to the global level. Moreover, multilateral organisations were considered as important funders if acknowledging the ethical dimension and acting accordingly (FG1, CJ, 637–49; FG2, SM + A, 842–51; FG3, LDA, 638–73).

*Orientation towards existing structures*
Present documents and mechanisms were mentioned by the participants to be used as references for a FGHP. Generally, it was stated that the availability of overarching, universal principles is important (FG1, CJ, 851–64; FG2, SC, 614–16; FG3, LDA, 303–09). Some of the existing documents are highly useful and have advanced for progress, while others require improvements. The major challenge in this regard refers to the lack of implementation of international agreements. As an example, Oriana mentioned the Cairo Platform for Action which was too vague and thus too ineffective (FG2, OLU, 635–42). She further criticised the quantitative focus of the SDGs and preceding MDGs, since this limits their potential to bring forward meaningful impact (FG2, OLU + A, 642–52). The participants demanded that without neglecting the local context, national governments must be pushed to adopt and act according to previously approved documents (FG1, CJ, 873–76, SKY, 889–92; FG2, OLU, 875–72). It was further highlighted that those agreements should not be considered in isolation but rather in a holistic way by recognising interlinkages with other frameworks (FG2, OLU, 652–58). Hence, the participants mentioned the following documents as useful for

a FGHP. Acknowledging the relevance of human rights, the Universal Declaration of Human Rights was frequently referred to as one of the most important global agreements (FG1, CJ, 862–64; FG2, OLU, 636–37; FG3, LDA, 302–04). FG1 also emphasised the significance of the Convention on the Elimination of All Forms of Discrimination Against Women, which, according to Jonathan "almost gives you a blueprint" (FG1, JC, 517) because of its comprehensive consideration of socio-economic determinants of health and rights (FG1, JC + A, 515–24, CJ + A, 857). Additionally, the Beijing Declaration and Platform for Action were considered "still relevant" (FG2, OLU, 879) (FG1, SKY, 883; FG2, OLU, 876–81). Moreover, national and regional agreements can serve as orientation for a FGHP and need to be taken into account for local implementation. Deborah mentioned the Maputo Protocol as one example (FG3, LDA, 303–08).

The participants also highlighted that meaningful international documents include participation and engagement of civil society, an aspect that is equally important for a FGHP (FG1, CJ + A, 876–81, SKY + A, 882–97).

## 6.8    Actors in FGHP

The focus group participants named relevant actors for a FGHP and elaborated on their role and responsibility. These have to be considered with regard to the previously depicted principles and components, as they are the responsible actors to adopt and implement a FGHP. Furthermore, questions of accountability were discussed. Importantly, the different actors should not be viewed in isolation. Rather, cooperation and participation are crucial for a purposeful FGHP and a high level of interlinkages between the actors exists.

*Community & civil society*
The significance of community and civil society was endorsed by all participants in the focus groups. They are regarded as the main actor for a FGHP and most relevant with respect to the subcode "Meaningful engagement". As Deborah stated, they are the "owners of this framework" (FG3, LDA, 383) because eventually, a FGHP serves to improve health and health equality for everyone in society.

Consistent with an intersectional understanding, community is not a homogenous group but rather includes various diverse actors. Referred to as most essential were community-based and grassroot-level organisations because of their local presence and context-specific knowledge (FG1, SKY + A, 657–63, JC, 697–99; FG2, SC, 460–62). Sandhya and Shubha mentioned community health workers and more specifically the role of Ashas in the Indian context as pivotal for primary health care (FG1, SKY, 670–73; FG2, SC, 462–80). Civil society and networks more broadly were also considered relevant, in particular for pushing feminist ideas (FG1, SKY + A, 701–07; FG2, SC, 536–38; OLU, 575–80; FG3, AN, 220–24). Much of the progress that has been achieved so far is due to the effort of communities (FG1, CJ, 864–66, 876–81). Throughout the discussions, the importance of feminist activists, thinkers, and movements was highlighted (FG1, CJ, 642–46, ER, 38–42; FG2, SM, 945–53; FG3, LDA, 601–03, 800–05). In this regard, Deborah stressed the contribution of "woman human rights defenders" (FG3, LDA, 254). Moreover, involving the whole community with "their different diversities and respect also their intersectionalities" (FG3, LDA, 272) was considered essential (FG1, CJ, 813–16; FG2, 503–05; FG3, AN, 228–35).

The engagement of community, and beyond that, the acknowledgement of this sector as key actor, was associated with improved health care and outcomes in the focus groups (FG2, SC + A, 225–32, OLU, 306–09). Contextualised knowledge and experiences ensure action based on what is genuinely needed and what challenges may occur (FG2, SM, 718–37; FG2, OLU, 439–45). As previously illustrated, the continuous meaningful engagement of community is pivotal for health equality and includes participation, listening, and shifting decisive power (FG1, MM; 375–77; FG2, SM, 707–17; FG3, LDA, 433–35). Communities and civil society are integral actors for empowering and educating the society and individuals. This also applies to the global context, where inclusion of various communities is important, while acknowledging different backgrounds (FG3, LDA, 452–67). Regarding FGHP, a bottom-up approach was identified as significant (FG2, SC, 481–83; FG3, 339–46). However, cooperation with the political level and an approach that "bring[s] bottom-up and top-down to each other" (FG3, AN, 338) was considered necessary (FG1, SE + A, 709–19, ER, 737–38). Consistently, national policymakers as actor in a FGHP are presented in the next section.

*National policymakers*
In addition to community and civil society, national policymakers were regarded as key actors for a FGHP. This implies states, governments, as well as individual policymakers. Their relevance derives from their impactful ability to decide over policies and laws concerning equality and health (FG3, LDA, 292–99, AN, 361–68). Acknowledging the model of the social determinants of health, the macrolevel strongly influences health. Participants of all focus groups identified that accountability for a FGHP resides at state level (FG1, SKY, 556–58; FG2, OLU, 567–68), with Charisse's words, "the states are the duty bearers" (FG1, CJ,

441–42). Adhering to the principle of democracy depicted in Section 6.6, governments and policymakers play a pivotal role (FG1, JC, 241–49; SE, 717–19). Political will and awareness are essential to enable change and improve health equality (FG2, OLU, 515–20). It is the state's responsibility to reduce the influence of the private sector in the health system (FG1, JC, 241–49). Because of the many current challenges linked to the political level, participants demanded a systemic change and transformation of political decision-making (FG2, SM + A, 397–407, OLU, 515–20, SC, 527–28). As frequently highlighted, participation and engagement of the community in the policy-making process is indispensable (FG2, OLU, 571–84; FG3, AN, 228–35, 335–38, 368–77). This implies a shift in power dynamics to ensure substantial transformation, also with regard to decoloniality (FG2, OLU, 656–61). National policymakers are also critical at global level, to foster intergovernmental exchange and collaboration (FG2, OLU, 876–82; FG3, LDA, 560–73).

*Multilateral organisations*
Community and national policymakers were considered the most significant actors for a FGHP. However, the participants also emphasised the relevance of multilateral organisations. As highlighted in Section 6.7, universal guidelines and global standards were regarded necessary. To develop and monitor those, multilateral organisations are required (FG1, CJ, 853–59; FG2, OLU, 313–17; FG3, AN, 662–65). Due to the global scope and anticipated application of a FGHP, the multilateral level—in particular UN organisations—should be considered (FG1, CJ, 646–48). Participants frequently referred to the WHO (FG1, ER, 328, JC, 695, CJ, 859; FG2, OLU, 313, SC, 592; FG3, AN, 650) and UN Women (FG3, AN, 650, LDA, 668). Global organisations have the potential to bring states together and to further establish linkages between all levels and actors involved (FG1, CJ, 872–76; FG3, LDA, 560–73, AN, 649–58). Moreover, they are influential actors because of their availability of resources, particularly for funding (FG3, AN, 650–51, 661–65, LDA, 669–73). In this respect, the participants noted that questions concerning accountability are important (FG1, ER, 322–32; FG2, SC + A, 588–94, 596–601). Due to their power, multilateral organisations must prove that they act meaningfully and ethically. Challenges exist with regard to the private sector and financial mechanisms at global level, particularly in the global health system (FG1, ER, 322–32, CJ, 637–42; FG2, SC + A, 588–94). However, if adhering to the principles outlined in Section 6.7, multilateral organisations can play a vital role in a FGHP.

## Academia

The role of academia in a FGHP can be derived from challenges concerning the subcode "Quantitative & biomedical focus" and the aspects illustrated in the subcode "Education within the health system". Academia is a minor actor in FGHP, but it was perceived as crucial with regard to education. Awa highlighted that academia and research must develop intersectional approaches and include reflexivity in their work (FG3, AN, 414–19). As the academic level is in charge of educating the future health workforce, consciousness about its responsibility and mechanisms to restructure the system are critical. Academia has the potential to foster change and improve healthcare and health outcomes (FG3, AN, 772–84). However, if the status quo remains and this responsibility is not fulfilled, adverse health impacts persist. The participants demanded universities to transform the current neoliberal, quantitative system, which neglects meaningful alternatives (FG1, MM + A, 380–84). Gendered and racist hierarchies within the health workforce are reinforced in this system. Acknowledging inherent power asymmetries and acting adequately was considered necessary (FG1, CJ, 649–56; FG2, OLU, 449–57; FG3, AN, 772–84). This shift also includes collaboration. Academic institutions tend to work in isolation. The participants discussed that the theoretical work should be better aligned with people on the ground (FG1, MM, 378–80; FG2, SM, 956–62). In this respect, academia should embark on a progressive transformation to advance health equality within a feminist global health policy (FG1, CJ, 642–46).

## Feminist economists

The subcode "Shift in funding" presented how to transform and adjust current funding mechanisms to align with the principles of a FGHP. In this respect, Jonathan introduced feminist economists as relevant actors. Where money comes from and what it is devoted to, has a profound impact on health. Health equality can be enhanced through a feminist approach to economy because of its "emphasis on equity and justice" (FG1, JC, 225). Feminist economists advocate for different perspectives on health economy that highly contrasts the current capitalistic system and its exploitative, oppressing characteristics (FG1, JC + A, 679–700, ER, 726–29). They facilitate power transformation since money is intertwined with power (ER, 897–906). Therefore, feminist economists represent an additional actor in a FGHP.

## Private sector

As presented in Section 6.1, the private sector was overwhelmingly associated with challenges in global health. Therefore, it was not considered as an integral actor in a FGHP. However, in the discussions references were made to the role of the private sector and what that encompasses. Participants emphasised that private sector actors must be held accountable and acknowledge their responsibility and—often detrimental—consequences of their actions (FG1, CJ, 192–200; FG2, SC + A, 585–88, OLU, 661–67). In the current global health system corporate actors are too powerful and influential, also with respect to national governments and multilateral institutions (FG1, JC, 217–21, ER, 322–27). As Oriana noticed "those are the ones that are ruling the the world right now" (FG2, OLU, 663–63). These power asymmetries have led to tremendous inequalities, which is why a power shift is pivotal. It was also noted that the private sector could still be involved to a lesser extent, if it adheres to fundamental values and principles and pursues good causes (FG1, CJ, 197–200, JC; 217–22). However, its role should mainly be supportive and limited, as the most integral actors are communities and national policymakers. As long as the adverse aspects of private sector engagement prevail, its inclusion should be treated with caution.

# Discussion

7

This research aimed to develop a framework for a feminist global health policy, informed by the focus group discussions and considerations of major contemporary challenges in global health. A synthesis of this framework is visualised in Figure 7.1 and serves as an overview to complement the comprehensive description provided in Chapter 6. The analysis reveals that considerations of power regimes, intersectionality, and knowledge paradigms are perceived as integral to the framework. Fundamental, universally applicable principles of human rights, equality, democracy, and decoloniality must be respected to achieve the objectives of health equality and reproductive justice for everyone. While adhering to global principles, the implementation of a FGHP is context-specific and acknowledges the respective SDOH. The results identified meaningful engagement of community and awareness raising at all levels as pivotal components of a FGHP. A shift in funding to feminist principles is considered as essential to ensure its financial feasibility and a departure from the current profit orientation fostered by the private sector. Adopting and implementing a FGHP denotes a radical transformation of the status quo. Key actors are community and civil society as well as national policymakers, followed by multilateral organisations. Academia and feminist economists can function as secondary actors who help sustain a feminist approach to global health policy.

In the following sections, these results are reflected upon with regard to the existing literature and discourse, their added value and implications, and the remaining gaps. This is followed by considerations of the methodological dimensions of this research.

H. Eger, *Feminist Global Health Policy*, BestMasters,
https://doi.org/10.1007/978-3-658-43497-7_7

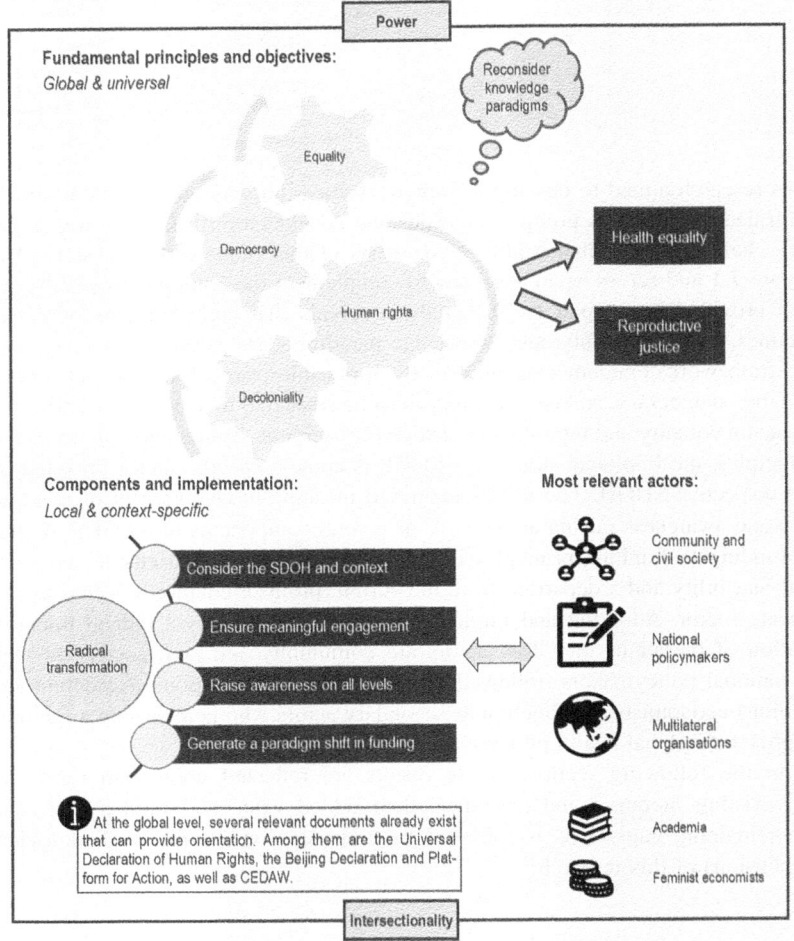

**FEMINIST GLOBAL HEALTH POLICY**
— Framework —

A feminist global health policy is a holistic, intersectional approach. Through recognising the influence of the socioeconomic-political level, power asymmetries and the resulting structural inequalities are challenged and transformed, leading to enhanced health and healthcare for everyone. Universal principles guide context-specific action, focusing on the most marginalised and ensuring participation and mutuality. Based on the human rights, a feminist global health policy is inherently decolonial.

Power

**Fundamental principles and objectives:**
*Global & universal*

Reconsider knowledge paradigms

Equality

Democracy

Human rights

Health equality

Reproductive justice

Decoloniality

**Components and implementation:**
*Local & context-specific*

Consider the SDOH and context

Ensure meaningful engagement

Radical transformation

Raise awareness on all levels

Generate a paradigm shift in funding

**Most relevant actors:**

Community and civil society

National policymakers

Multilateral organisations

At the global level, several relevant documents already exist that can provide orientation. Among them are the Universal Declaration of Human Rights, the Beijing Declaration and Platform for Action, as well as CEDAW.

Academia

Feminist economists

Intersectionality

**Fig. 7.1**  Synthesis of a feminist global health policy

## 7.1    Discussion of the findings

*Orientation towards existing structures*

This research sought to reference and build upon relevant existing global agreements, which are described in Section 3.1 and emphasised by the participants in the FGDs. In this regard, the principles and components of a FGHP identified through this research are aligned with and already promoted in established agreements, most prominently the Universal Declaration of Human Rights and CEDAW, as well as the Beijing Declaration and Platform for Action. Despite limitations due to the use of exclusively quantitative indicators to measure progress on the SDGs, the objectives of the 2030 Agenda and in particular of SDGs 3, 5, and 10 (on health, gender equality, and reduced inequalities respectively) also confirm to the findings on FGHP. Hence, these globally established agreements provide orientation when adopting a FGHP. Further alignment and consistence with the existing state of the literature and discourse is evident.

*Feminist approaches to policy*

In 2021, the Centre for Feminist Foreign Policy (CFFP) published a policy briefing on feminist global health policy (CFFP, 2021). Their policy recommendations for implementing a FGHP to achieve health equality share considerable similarities to the results of the present study. In line with the current findings, the CFFP (2021) demands a transformation of power, including rethinking financial flows, with specific recommendations for the global and the local level. A focus on equality (also within the global health realm), marginalised groups, and SRHR is evident throughout the briefing. Harmful norms and their manifestations are to be recognised and addressed. Consistent with the results of this research, a FGHP is presented as an inherently holistic, intersectional, and decolonial approach (CFFP, 2021). Similar principles and priorities are also emphasised in an article on feminist global health by Davies and colleagues (2019). These publications closely correspond to the reported findings of this research, due to the adherence to intersectional feminist principles. The added value provided by the findings of this study derives from the profound reflections on contemporary challenges. Furthermore, this framework for a FGHP combines universal principles, which are referenced in the current discourse, with recommendations for local implementation, thus respecting the necessity for context-specific adaptation.

The policy fields of foreign policy, so-called development policy[1], and global health policy are closely interlinked (Bernarding et al., 2021; Gunda-Werner-Institut et al., 2022; VENRO, 2022). Consequently, they should not be understood in isolation. Rather, intersectoral exchange should be encouraged and coherent strategies across these policy fields should be promoted. Feminist approaches to politics have become increasingly prominent in recent years, most notably in foreign policy and global cooperation policy. Feminist global health policy is in comparison still in its infancy, but distinct parallels can be drawn to more established feminist policy fields. In this regard, it is relevant to consider the extent to which the framework for a FGHP presented as the outcome of this research strongly aligns with the literature on other feminist policies.

For example, in the CFFP manifesto for a feminist foreign policy such an approach is outlined as genuinely intersectional, decolonial, transformative, and human-rights centred (Bernarding et al., 2021). The objective of a feminist foreign policy is the termination of inequalities and discrimination. Acknowledging and ensuring the participation of civil society is considered crucial. The same components are emphasised in a recent publication by 18 German civil society organisations on feminist foreign policy (Gunda-Werner-Institut et al., 2022). The transformative character is regarded as necessary to dismantle existing patriarchal structures and shifting power to communities. This includes a change in financial structures. In an article linking feminist foreign policy to global health, Irwin (2019) highlights the importance of considering implementation from the onset, i.e. policy formulation—an aspect this research project specifically aims to address. Close parallels exist as well with a publication by the umbrella organisation for humanitarian NGOs in Germany VENRO (2022) about feminist global cooperation policy. The underlying principles are the same as mentioned previously. Moreover, the need to include and strengthen civil society is endorsed, as well as the necessity to rethink power dynamics. Persisting (colonial, patriarchal) perceptions have to be questioned to enable systemic change (VENRO, 2022). Accordingly, the presented framework for a FGHP closely relates to existing feminist approaches to foreign policy and global cooperation policy. This reinforces the relevance of the current findings and the potential to align a FGHP with other feminist policy approaches. It remains to be seen—with hope—whether feminist global health policy will be the next policy field to enter the mainstream debate.

---

[1] The use of the term "development" originates from a colonial mindset. Feminist approaches want to overcome this connotation by introducing the term "feminist global cooperation policy" (Heinrich-Böll-Stiftung & Fair Share, 2022).

In addition to explicitly feminist policies, the results identified can be compared to evidence on gender and health equality more broadly, as feminist approaches to global health are not necessarily always labelled as such.

*Health equality and universal principles*
The interlinkage between human rights and equality and their significance for global health is well established and was emphasised in the FGDs. Khosla and colleagues (2022) reinforce that "gender equality is necessary for health as a human right" (p. 2) and highlight the political imperative to fulfil these rights." Safaei (2012) further confirms the correlation between human rights, democracy, and women's health. Equality is also a prerequisite for the progressive decolonisation of global health. The findings from the FGDs suggest that achieving genuine decoloniality requires a systemic transformation, corresponding to the positions of Abimbola and Pai (2020) and Büyüm and colleagues (2020). The necessity of contextualised political action respecting the SDOH—a critical component in the elaborated framework—is also evident in the literature. This understanding aligns with the conceptual framework on the SDOH by Solar and Irwin (2010) (Figure 5.1), which highlights the relevance of acknowledging the SDOH and the impact of the socioeconomic-political context and globalisation on health equality and health. Several publications provide recommendations for incorporating considerations of gender and health equality into policy processes. For instance, Dhatt and Pley (2021) and Heymann and colleagues (2019) suggest implementing gender-transformative programmes to reduce gender inequality and improve health. Consistent with an intersectional approach and the recognition of multiple interlinkages, multisectoral action beyond the health sector is mentioned as crucial element for sustainable change, reflecting the concept of health in all policies (CFFP, 2021; Gupta et al., 2019; Heymann et al., 2019; Solar & Irwin, 2010). Another focal point for meaningful change is monitoring (Heymann et al., 2019; Sridharan et al., 2016). In this respect, a FGHP must be closely monitored and evaluation should be ongoing rather than ceasing after implementation.

The existing literature often provides more detailed recommendations about specific aspects of the health system. The objective of this research was to develop an overarching global framework that could be applied to multiple areas of concern, i.e. a framework that elaborates a set of cross-cutting principles and components, which when respected could lead to improvements across various sectors and contexts. Due to this global and universal scope, examples were not provided or discussed in detail in the focus groups. Publications that do focus on narrower research topics provide context- or topic-specific recommendations that resonate with the examples presented in Section 2.2.2. Accordingly, these studies constitute a coherent continuation of the aforementioned findings and demonstrate the positive impacts of the proposed FGHP framework when applied to certain areas.

### Healthcare system

As endorsed in the FGDs, health equality can only be achieved by improved healthcare and access. Hay and colleagues (2019) as well as Dhatt and Pley (2021) confirm the findings that health systems should reflect intersectionality and respond to the needs of all people, with a focus on marginalised groups. Progressive achievement of UHC requires that healthcare is affordable, accessible, available, and of decent quality (Dhatt & Pley, 2021; Hay et al., 2019). With its structural, intersectional approach, a FGHP can support efforts to mitigate adverse health impacts that derive from the gendered pathways to health identified by Heise and colleagues (2019). In accordance with findings of the present study, a precondition for more just health systems is to address underlying inequalities, as Hay and colleagues (2019) note in a study from the Lancet Series on gender equality, norms, and health. With regard to the fulfilment of SRHR, the report of the Guttmacher–Lancet Commission by Starrs and colleagues (2018) provide very similar recommendations to those identified in this research, e.g. acknowledging the significance of the SDOH as well as the need for policy change. They further emphasise the interconnectedness of reproductive justice with gender and health equality (Starrs et al., 2018).

Intersectional inequalities in the health workforce, resulting from patriarchy, capitalism, and racism, were highlighted in the focus groups. In their policy recommendations to achieve UHC and gender equality, Sen and colleagues (2020) confirm the need to recognise and ensure labour rights of the health workforce and address gendered inequalities. Consistently, Gupta and colleagues (2019) advocate for a reform of the health workforce and working conditions to eliminate restrictive gender norms that uphold inequalities. Health workers should have equal opportunities to pursue their career, irrespective of gender, race, class, and further determinants (Hay et al., 2019). Several publications highlight the request for fair representation on political and leadership level. While statements in the FGDs revealed the importance of meaningful engagement and a transformation of power—which are requirements for (political) representation—specific recommendations for "substantive representation" (Davies et al., 2019, p. 601) and considerations on equal leadership opportunities within global health were not mentioned. Heymann and colleagues (2019) reaffirm the importance of political representation of women to foster gender equality and improve health outcomes. Regarding global health organisations, Newman and colleagues (2017) demand gender-equal composition of staff to strengthen leadership and representation. However, Herten-Crabb and Davies (2020) note that women do not equal feminism and therefore embodying feminist principles is most relevant regardless of gender. In accordance with intersectional gender analysis, this should be extended to include further marginalised groups.

The limitations of quantitative data for public and global health was another important issue identified by participants in the FGDs and through the review of literature. Consistent with these findings, Khosla and colleagues (2022) criticise the narrow biomedical and quantitative scope that continues to dominate in global health and emphasise the importance of context for purposeful policies (Khosla et al., 2022). The examples presented in Section 2.2.2 demonstrate the lack of gender-equitable research and its impact on health. In accordance, Gupta and colleagues (2019) demand gender-responsive data systems for "filling gaps in data and eliminating gender bias in research" (Gupta et al., 2019, p. 2551). The CFFP (2021) also calls for diversification of research, in particular with a focus on marginalised groups and SRHR. The demand for more comprehensive data is reflected in the current results, in accordance with findings from Heidari and Doyle (2020).

### *Meaningful engagement and relevant actors*
Meaningfully engaging the community and ensuring accountability at the political level were regarded in the FGDs as pivotal for a FGHP. As Audre Lorde remarked, "Without community there is no liberation." (Lorde, 1984, p. 112). This perspective is reaffirmed by multiple studies. Heymann and colleagues (2019) examined the importance of social participation and raising awareness to dismantle power relations and restrictive gender norms, as a means to reduce gender inequality and improve health outcomes. Concordantly, Gupta and colleagues (2019) identified civil society organisations as crucial actors—when adequately and sustainably funded. This aspect is reiterated by Fulu and colleagues (2021) with particular reference to feminist movements. Solar and Irwin (2010) likewise highlight the significance of including civil society, as well as "the empowerment of affected communities to become active protagonists in shaping their own health." (p. 58). Autonomy and self-determination, inherent to empowerment, are critical to improve health equality and health. Participation of affected and marginalised people at political level is therefore required. Consistent with findings of this research, Solar and Irwin (2010) regard national policymakers as primarily accountable for this integration: it is their responsibility to ensure meaningful participation within the policy process. This position is equally maintained by Gupta and colleagues (2019) who advocate for enhanced accountability

mechanisms. Transparency and accountability are furthermore regarded as essential to decolonise global health (Khan et al., 2021). The critical importance of the political level for health (equality) is frequently noted, due to its competence to develop and adopt laws and policies. As mentioned by Khosla and colleagues (2022) "Laws matter as much as medicine" (p. 2). In accordance with statements in the focus groups, Heymann and colleagues (2019) highlight the potential of laws and policies to enhance health and gender equality, at national as well as global level. For example, the EU research project SOPHIE clearly demonstrated the positive impact of gender-sensitive policies on gender equality and health (Palència et al., 2017).

### *Multilateral organisations and financial mechanisms*
In addition to the national level, the global level is also regarded as central—in relevant literature as well as by participants in the FGDs. In 2008, the Commission on the Social Determinants of Health (CSDH, 2008) pointed to the necessity to strengthen the WHO and its leadership regarding action on the SDOH. Fourteen years later, this continues to be pertinent. For example, with Khosla and colleagues (2022) calling for structural change of the UN family, including less dependence on external actors and more global authority. Irwin (2019) argues that feminist policies also serve to hold multilateral organisations accountable to agreed-upon commitments to equality. In this regard, adequate funding of these institutions is crucial, consistent with the perspective of Heymann and colleagues (2019), who reaffirm the significance of funding for gender and health equality. Herten-Crabb and Davies (2020) advocate for the WHO to adopt an explicitly "feminist economic agenda" (p. 1018). According to the authors this implies a focus on intersectionality and power—particularly on power asymmetries between genders as well as states—and the recognition of the SDOH in economic decisions. Such an approach could potentially improve continuous gendered and intersectional inequalities faced by the health workforce. It further entails refraining from austerity measures that adversely affect public health expenditures (Herten-Crabb & Davies, 2020). This aligns with the identified request for a shift to feminist funding in the present analysis.

The insistence on responsible action at global level, including regarding financial structures, is also expressed in the global social policy literature. Most notably, Deacon (2007) elaborates that global social policy, of which global health policy is a part, is concerned with *Redistribution, Regulation,* and *Rights.* Redistribution promotes equality within society. At global level, redistributive mechanisms adhere to a decolonial approach since the Global North has an obligation to the Global South. Redistribution could therefore foster global equality.

This aligns with the results of this analysis, which promote feminist approaches to economy and the principle of decoloniality. Regulation is another focal point, considering the influence of the private sector and the resulting weakness of governments. Deacon (2007) refers to multiple areas of concern, specifically including the lack of global regulation of healthcare. This challenge was likewise mentioned in the focus groups and the results indicate the need for greater regulation by national policymakers as well as multilateral organisations. Furthermore, Deacon (2007) highlights the importance of human rights and their fulfilment, an aspect equally endorsed in this study as already described. The presented FGHP framework therefore appears to be consistent with priorities and principles inherent to global social policy.

### Additional determinants and intersectionality

The present research focuses in particular on the structural determinants gender, race, class, and their implications on health. However, as the elaborated framework for a FGHP is based on the analysis of power and an intersectional understanding, it can be applied to diverse determinants and systems of oppression. Additional intersecting determinants of relevance can be identified in the literature, most notably related to sexuality with regard to health (e.g. Alencar Albuquerque et al., 2016; Medina-Martínez et al., 2021; Wilson & Cariola, 2020). Profound consideration of how these aspects can be considered for a FGHP is an important avenue for further empirical research. The significance of climate justice and planetary health for a FGHP is one priority area for which further in-depth examination is essential, including in relation to the abovementioned issues and questions. The interlinkage between health and gender equality and climate change are well recognised (e.g. WHO, 2014). Climate change constitutes one of the major cotemporary challenges for global health and human development. The direct and indirect health impacts of climate change are not distributed equally, but are highly gendered and tend to impact marginalised people the most (Barre et al., 2022; Habtezion, 2016; WHO, 2014). In this regard, women face worse outcomes than men, often related to intersecting inequalities based on social class. These inequalities are evident within as well as between countries, revealing the influence of colonial structures. Therefore, intersectionality and structural power dimensions are equally important considering climate change (Deivanayagam et al., 2022; Habtezion, 2016; WHO, 2014). Deivanayagam and colleagues (2022) emphasise the continuous impacts of colonialism on climate and health and highlight adverse health effects of racism, endorsed by climate change at national and global level. The scope of coloniality and racism, intersecting with capitalism and patriarchy, becomes evident when looking at global causes for climate change. Hickel (2022) analysed that Global North countries account for 92 % of excess global $CO^2$ emissions, while people in the Global South are most affected by detrimental health outcomes. Mechanisms to address climate change and its implications must be centred on equality and equity and guided by social justice. This includes participatory approaches and the involvement of lived experiences (Barre et al., 2022; Deivanayagam et al., 2022; WHO, 2014). Corresponding interventions are identified, for instance the "Gender Just Climate Solutions" provided by the Women and Gender Constituency (Barre et al., 2022). Climate change was not explicitly mentioned in the FGDs, however the recommendations for action on climate change align with the FGHP framework and reflect universal principles. Further consideration is needed about how a FGHP can be applied to and of value in addressing issues related to planetary health and climate justice.

*Overarching contribution of this study and areas for future research*
This research project constitutes a comprehensive, interdisciplinary effort to elaborate a framework for feminist global health policy. Universal principles as well as components for context-specific implementation are identified with reference to relevant actors and their accountability. Thus, the framework establishes a link between the global and local level. The research interest was guided by the idea—and ideal—of a feminist approach towards global health policy, a somewhat utopian and aspirational vision which provides a space for imagination and reflection. Inspired by bell hooks' words "What we cannot imagine cannot come into being." (hooks, 2001, p. 14), this study intended to stimulate and provoke reconsiderations of power dynamics and epistemologies. This research offers decisive added value as the foundation of the framework is deeply embedded in considerations of intersectionality, power relations, and knowledge paradigms. By placing power in the centre of the FGHP framework, a comprehensive understanding of intersectionality and structural roots of inequalities is fostered. While this research focused on the structural determinants of gender, race, and class, the framework is not exclusive of considering further determinants and their interlinkages. The embodiment of an intersectional approach highlights both the interconnectedness of inequalities and the importance of collaboration between social movements to enable radical transformation—while acknowledging the complexity of this endeavour and the rejection of isolated solutions. The relevance of "pluriversality" (FG1, ER, 767) identified in the analysis—with regard to alternatives, but also feminist, intersectional, and decolonial approaches—aligns with the concept of the *mosaic left* by Urban (2009). Originally intended as a response to capitalistic power structures, this concept can be applied more broadly to any form of critical social movement. Urban (2009) argues that different actors must

come together and cooperate for the common good. Although endeavours and intentions of the individuals may differ, they pursue the same goals. Therefore, building alliances is important. This is what Urban (2009) refers to as mosaic left. The present research project can also be considered from this perspective—the intention is not to generate one singular, comprehensive solution, it should rather be perceived as a mosaic piece on the path to health equality, reproductive justice, and power transformation.

This further reflects the choice of a postmodern epistemology. Since postmodernism presumes that reality is shaped by subjective perceptions, the identification of one universal solution was not intended, but to provide an adaptable and flexible instrument. The intention is to ensure adherence to mutually agreed universal principles, while facilitating needs-based, context-specific implementation to eventually improve the health of all people. The application of feminist methods and underlying considerations about ontology, epistemology, and methodology are mirrored in the findings of this study. They are subject of discussion in Section 7.2.

As with all research projects, several questions remained unanswered in this study. The presented results identified principles and components for a meaningful implementation of a FGHP. However, power must be shifted for sustainable change. This aspect requires further considerations. Knowledge and ideas about implementing policies already exist, but genuine action is still lacking. While this study provides important recommendations, further action-based research on contextual implementation is needed to turn the imagination space into action. Shifting power also requires sensitisation of those already in power about the significance of transferring power for the benefit of all people. How can people in power be reached, educated, and convinced? How to proceed in non-democratic contexts? Changing power systems further demands intensive reflections on power itself, as well as on further definitions and concepts, e.g. global health and feminism. Established definitions often do not reflect the influence of power regimes, mainly coloniality and patriarchy, that is embedded in knowledge paradigms. In light of the emergence of anti-feminist movements around the world, questions arise of how to strengthen feminist movements. How can a space of collaboration and allyship for the common good be created, that entails different intentions and interests, as proposed by the concept of the mosaic left?

## 7.2    Methodological Discussion

In this subchapter the methodology described in Chapter 5 is critically reflected upon in terms of strengths and limitations. As part of the practice of reflexivity, it is essential to recognise how the positionality and subjectivity of the researcher (see Section 5.6) influence the results. A postmodern epistemology, which underpins this research, considers subjectivity not as a deficit but rather unavoidable as the world is perceived as socially constructed. Acknowledging positionality takes into account this complexity and the notion of multiple subjective truths rather than one objective reality. Olmos-Vega and colleagues (2022) emphasise the contribution of reflexivity by stating:

> Embrace your subjectivity; abandon objectivity as a foundational goal and embrace the power of your subjectivity through meaningful reflexivity practices. Reflexivity is not a limitation; it is an asset in your research. (Olmos-Vega et al., 2022, p. 9)

The extent to which reflexivity was adopted meaningfully in this research is considered, in addition to a critical reflection of how this research "fulfils feminist objectives" (Wilkinson, 1988, p. 495).

### *Strengths*
The interdisciplinary approach inherent to this research presents a major strength. This interdisciplinary study demonstrates interlinkages between the fields of global (public) health and political science. The study highlights not only the necessity to consider the complementary insights of both disciplinary perspectives, but the specific added value generated by this interdisciplinary lens when applied to the topic of feminist global health policy. Combining evidence and methods from the two disciplines results in insights and outcomes that are more than the sum of their parts. Including feminist perspectives further reinforces interdisciplinarity. The demand for interdisciplinary research on health inequalities and the SDOH is highlighted in the literature (e.g. Kivits et al., 2019). Moreover, participatory approaches are essential for interdisciplinary research (Aboelela et al., 2007; Padberg, 2014). In this regard, this study is interdisciplinary on two levels: Firstly, in terms of the background of the researcher, who unites the disciplines of public health and political science, and secondly, in terms of employing a participatory approach involving actors from a variety of backgrounds.

The inclusion of multiple standpoints is also essential for an intersectional approach, to acknowledge interlinked determinants, privileges, and oppression. Intersectionality requires interdisciplinary research and the intersectional approach itself is another strength of this study (Dill & Kohlman, 2012). An intersectional gender analysis was conducted that seeks to consider the structural determinants of gender, race, class, and their interconnectedness. While gender was the primary entry point and focus, all aspects were considered from an intersectional perspective (WHO, 2020). According to the WHO (2020) categorisation, this research counts as gender-transformative, since power regimes and resulting structural (gendered) inequalities are addressed and challenged. Furthermore, this research is intended to foster transformation of global health policy towards equality.

The fundamental methodological principles of this research have proven to be very valuable. The application of feminist methods facilitated a decolonial, participatory approach. Emphasis on participation supported the reduction of power hierarchies within the research process and represents a great advantage for the results. Equally meaningful was the decision for a postmodern epistemology. Underlying presumptions of postmodernism (depicted in Chapter 5) were mirrored in the results. Questions regarding what counts as knowledge and the rejection of a singular truth were reflected in the focus group discussions, enhancing a postmodern understanding. Embedded in postmodernism is the perception of a socially constructed world, which relates to the concepts of gender, race, and class. The choice of focus groups as the methodological approach for data collection adequately aligns with postmodernism and feminist principles as multiple standpoints were included and listened to. Participants were diverse in terms of their geographical location and their scope of action, backgrounds, and experiences. The participatory approach enabled meaningful engagement of participants within the process and made them—and community more broadly—"owners of this framework" (FG3, LDA, 383). The appropriateness of focus groups as data collection instrument was also highlighted by the participants themselves (e.g. FG1, MM+A, 1084–87; JC+A, 1089–93). Consistent with the literature, the participants thus benefitted from the exchange. Exploitation common in other forms of research could be reduced (Lamnek & Krell, 2016). Power hierarchies were dismantled and context and subjectivity considered. As the researcher acted as moderator and sought to remain in the background, the focus was on the participants, in alignment with feminist research methods and objectives (Bryman, 2016; Wilkinson, 1999). Despite diverse backgrounds and experiences, similarities and agreements within and across the three focus groups were identified. The dynamic and flexibility of focus groups allowed for new insights and vivid discussions, which would not necessarily have emerged in individual interviews (Bryman, 2016; Lamnek & Krell, 2016). Online focus groups in particular feature a higher level of accessibility: participants could attend irrespective of their geographical location without the need to travel and free of costs. In this regard, it is less time-consuming for the participants and they can join from home or work, i.e. in a familiar environment (Bryman, 2016). This research project would have not been feasible without using online focus groups due to the broad geographical scope. It is a great added value of this study to involve and connect people and perspectives from all over the world to discuss a FGHP.

This research further fulfils most of the quality criteria proposed by Tracy (2010) for qualitative research, described in Section 5.1.4. The topic of feminist global health policy presents a relevant, interesting, and significant topic and can thus be considered as *worthy*. The criterion of *rich rigor* is achieved by including a variety of perspectives in the focus groups and emphasising intersectionality. Complex constructs were considered prior to data collection as well as in the analysis. According to Tracy (2010) *sincerity* can be reached by reflexivity of the researcher and providing transparency about methods and challenges. The latter will be subject of discussion subsequently. Reflexivity was practiced throughout the research process, particularly by including reflexive writing in the form of memos after the focus group discussions and member reflection (Olmos-Vega et al., 2022). Further information about reflexivity and positionality of the researcher can be obtained from Sections 5.6 and 7.2. These mechanisms also enhance the *credibility* of the research. This criterion is further respected by including multiple standpoints and non-verbal interactions, consistent with Tracy's (2010) recommendations. The impact of this research on the audience, in line with the criterion *resonance*, remains to be seen. However, a degree of transferability of the findings can be assumed since different contexts and perspectives were included. The participants expressed that they appreciated the exchange and felt inspired by the discussions (e.g. FG1, JC, 1090–93). Furthermore, the framework is designed for context-specific adaption. In this regard, this research is intended to provide a *significant contribution*, for researchers as well as for practitioners and politicians, as the results encourage a transformation of policy-making. *Ethical* considerations are presented in Section 5.7 and were considered throughout the research, in particular to adhere to feminist principles. This study can be considered as "*meaningfully coherent*" (Tracy, 2010, p. 848) because the background, methods, and results align very well with the intended objective and offer a high degree of consistency. Accordingly, this research provides a strong degree of quality with respect to the criteria introduced by Tracy (2010).

### Limitations

Notwithstanding the abovementioned strengths, some important limitations of this study need to be acknowledged.

While this study embraces an interdisciplinary approach, the research was not conducted by an interdisciplinary team, but by a single researcher. While both disciplines, public health and political science, were combined, knowledge and experience of only one researcher were incorporated. This limits interdisciplinarity, which is enhanced by team work (Aboelela et al., 2007).

Secondly, the scope of the participatory approach was by necessity limited. In contrast to comprehensive participatory research approaches, inclusion and cooperation was only considered for the results, rather than the whole research process. The research question and methodology were conceptualised by the researcher, who also analysed the outcomes and interpreted the findings. According to Wright (2021), participation is ideally incorporated from the beginning and at every stage of research. Genuine participation is a valuable mechanism to reduce power hierarchies and avoid exploitation. However, this is a highly intense, time-consuming endeavour—for both, the researcher as well as participants. This was not feasible within the timeframe of a master's thesis and could also lead to overstretching the resources of—and thus exploiting—the participants. Finding a balance between genuine participation and not demanding too much energy, time, and effort from the participants was a challenge of this research. Consistent with feminist principles, participation was endorsed, although the researcher was reluctant to require too much commitment since the results are nonetheless primarily used for her master's thesis. In this regard, a compromise between participation and respecting the time expenditure of the participants was sought.

The practice of reflexivity applied in this research must also be critically reflected upon. The importance of reflexivity, particularly for qualitative health and feminist research, is depicted previously (e.g. Olmos-Vega et al., 2022; Wilkinson, 1988). In addition to the lack of an interdisciplinary team in this research, collaborative reflexivity could not be genuinely applied. However, it was considered by adopting member reflection (Olmos-Vega et al., 2022). The influence of the researcher's positionality could have been highlighted more throughout the research and analysis. The same accounts for the context and positionality of the participants. Due to the limited scope of a master's thesis, these aspects were not referred to in great detail. Information about the participants can be obtained from Table 5.1. Regarding the researcher's positionality, indicated in Section 5.6, not all power hierarchies could be dismantled during the research process. The decision for focus groups and a participatory approach reduced power asymmetries. However, that did not alter the fact that the principal researcher is a privileged white, well-educated, middle-class woman from a Global North country. The presented results should therefore be interpreted in consideration of this positionality. Moreover, the subjectivity of the participants determined the results, as anticipated when conducting focus groups based on a postmodern epistemology. This implies that a different group composition could have resulted in divergent outcomes (Lamnek & Krell, 2016). Contextualisation and acknowledgment of a socially constructed world does not constitute a disadvantage, yet should be reflected when considering the results. To further discuss and develop the FGHP framework, it would be interesting to conduct a fourth focus group with participants from all previous groups. This group would not comply with the criterion of homogeneity. However, not all participants could easily be allocated to one of the focus groups conducted because of their multiple affiliations. This emphasises the complexity of the social world as well as intersecting identities. It also raises the questions of how many focus groups and participants are adequate, considering that saturation is not an anticipated criterion in a postmodern perspective. Rather, this research can be understood as providing insights for a continuing process that is not completed with this work.

Some specific limitations should also be mentioned regarding the conduct of focus groups. Focus groups are a time-consuming process, in terms of both the coordination in advance as well as for the analysis, while the scope of this research needed to comply with the regulations of a master's thesis (Bryman, 2016). The non-response rate for focus groups is considerably high and was two-thirds in this study. Such an approach therefore required extensive preparation. The inclusion and exclusion criteria also reflect some limitations. The focus groups had to proceed in English (as the contemporary international *lingua franca*), to ensure communication and mutual understanding between participants. However, this can be regarded as a shortcoming with respect to persisting coloniality in global health. Individuals not proficient in English were excluded. Such an approach risks inadvertently excluding or bypassing of meaningful contributions of community members and people with lived experiences. In addition, only those with access to a stable internet connection could attend, which further excluded potential participants (Bryman, 2016). Connectivity issues also caused difficulties during the focus groups. One participant was unable to attend FG2 as scheduled due to a power outage. However, this problem was solved by conducting an additional third focus group. Non-attendance was equally a challenge in FG3. While the difficulties in FG2 were explained and solved, one participant did not attend FG3 without notice. Consequently, FG3 only consisted of two participants and the moderator. While more attendees would have stimulated the discussion in FG3, valuable insights were nevertheless generated, including some consistent with FG1 and FG2, as well as new considerations being raised. The smaller group size led to longer individual talking time that provided meaningful contributions.

Interaction and non-verbal communication were considered, constituting a strength of this research. The online format led to some limitations. Interaction can be captured more extensively in face-to-face focus groups. It is also more difficult in an online setting to establish a familiar atmosphere between previously unknown participants (Bryman, 2016). This can also be regarded as a limitation in the quality criterion *rich rigor* according to Tracy (2010). The context and positionality of the participants could have been more prominent in the analysis, for example by including thick description. A detailed description of the context of the focus groups and participants and the analysis of more complex data could have further enhanced the criterion *credibility* (Tracy, 2010). Since such an approach is very demanding for the participants and the researcher, it was not feasible within the scope of this thesis.

In summary, and in light of the strengths and limitations of this research, the FGHP framework provides a meaningful contribution and insights. Rather than considering the findings as a completed project, they should be understood as a stimulus for further elaboration. As Shubha noted, the presented framework should be perceived as

> something that allows people to take what they want, add, eject, shape, reshape, you know. [...] Like clay where you can keep moulding and re-moulding it. (FG2, SC, 631–34)

## 7.3   Recommendations

Based on the theoretical background (Chapter 2), the results of this study (Chapter 6), and the discussion, including the identified gaps (Section 7.1), recommendations for policymakers and researchers are provided in Table 7.1. The elaborated FGHP framework is intended to serve as a point of reference—for concrete political action as well as for further research. This implies, on the one hand, the consideration and implementation of the framework and, on the other hand, its continuous development and reflection. With regard to intersectionality and contextualisation, the recommendations should not be understood in isolation. As indicated by the results, it is pivotal for researchers, policymakers, and community members to cooperate for structural changes and sustainable alternatives. The inclusion, participation, and empowerment of community must always be considered. Accordingly, any overlaps between recommendations for policymakers and researchers is encouraged.

**Table 7.1** Recommendations for policymakers and researchers

| Recommendations | | |
|---|---|---|
| **Policymakers** | | **Research** |
| **Multilateral** | **National** | |
| ➢ Reflect on privileges (at individual & institutional level) | | ➢ Practice reflexivity: Reflect on positionality and the effects on research |
| ➢ Reflect and address power regimes (at institutional & societal level) | | |
| ➢ Enable a shift in power:<br>  ○ Meaningfully include community & civil society in all processes<br>  ○ Apply participatory approaches<br>  ○ Work in cooperation<br>  ○ Listen to people and their lived experience<br>  ○ Acknowledge diversity<br>  ○ Transform rhetoric into action | | ➢ Use the present framework for future research<br>  ○ Extent or adjust the framework<br>  ○ Research the feasibility of the framework, e.g. implementation for a specific context or topic |
| | | ➢ Apply feminist research methods and reduce power imbalances in the research process |
| ➢ Respect human rights and act accordingly | | ➢ Adopt more holistic approaches within global health research |
| ➢ Engage with new approaches that transcend the status quo | | |
| ➢ Adopt feminist principles and recognise that gender and feminism are not synonymous with women | | ➢ Apply research tools that can be used to study intersectionality in its complexity, do not rely on an exclusively quantitative approach |
| ➢ Centre on intersectionality:<br>  ○ Acknowledge multiple power asymmetries and resulting implications for health<br>  ○ Do not neglect marginalised people | | ➢ Conduct participatory research:<br>  ○ Research for the people affected and not for yourself / your career<br>  ○ Include the community at all stages, engage with the people meaningfully<br>  ○ Needs-based, decolonial orientation |
| ➢ Apply intersectional gender analysis for policies, laws, programmes, interventions | | |
| ➢ Encourage intersectoral work & the Health in all policies approach | | ➢ Appreciate lived experience and other sources of evidence |
| ➢ Prioritise achieving health equality & reproductive justice by focusing on structural inequalities and the SDOH | | |

(continued)

**Table 7.1** (continued)

| Recommendations | | Research |
|---|---|---|
| **Policymakers** | | |
| **Multilateral** | **National** | |
| ➤ Restrict the influence of the private sector & profit orientation in health significantly | | ➤ In the academic context:<br>○ Adjust the curriculum for health workers<br>○ Teach in accordance with a FGHP |
| ➤ Change funding for global/public health<br>○ Apply feminist economist principles<br>○ Provide more funding for holistic, horizontal programmes that address structural causes<br>○ Accept and encourage a broader evidence base alongside quantitative indicators for funded projects<br>○ Provide funding in cooperation with the education sector for awareness raising & sensitisation projects | | |
| ➤ Reinforce globally established agreements | ➤ Fulfil democratic values | |
| ➤ Elaborate a globally applicable FGHP based on the presented framework | ➤ Adhere to global agreements, including a globally agreed FGHP | |
| ➤ Provide space for international exchange | ➤ Acknowledge accountability to the population | |
| ➤ Operate as watchdog, ensure effective monitoring and accountability mechanisms | ➤ Transfer agreements into action through meaningful implement-tation based on this framework | |
| ➤ Advance decolonial approaches | ➤ Ensure healthcare is affordable, accessible, available & of high quality | |
| ➤ Strengthen the UN and related organisations, particularly regarding more (financial) independence & authority | ➤ Ensure adequate renumeration for the health workforce and eliminate gender & other inequalities therein | |
| ➤ Reinforce the WHO to live up to its mandate and the promise of health for all, including health equality and reproductive justice | | |
| ➤ Reconsider global spending for health<br>○ Advance global redistribution mechanisms<br>○ Reject the colonial "donor-aid" mentality | | |

# Conclusion

8

In this thesis the research question "How can a feminist approach to global health policy be meaningfully implemented to reduce health inequalities?" has been examined. The elaborated framework for a feminist global health policy serves as guidance for policymakers, practitioners, and communities, as well as for further research. It is based on an intersectional understanding that is centred on power (Hill Collins, 2019). Four main universal principles—human rights, equality, democracy, decoloniality—were identified to guide a FGHP towards health equality and reproductive justice (Figure 7.1). The framework is generated to link the global with the local level by allowing for context-specific adaptation while respecting universal principles. Implementation must be based on the respective needs. Accordingly, it is imperative for a FGHP to meaningfully engage the people concerned. In this regard, community is considered as the most important actor (FG3, LDA, 379–84). Structurally embedded power asymmetries, determining inequalities, indicate that accountability remains at political level (FG1, CJ, 441–42; Solar & Irwin, 2010). Feminist global health policy concerns politics as much as it concerns health. It is laws and policies that influence the structural determinants of health, among them gender, race, and class. Consequently, health inequalities, caused by structural inequities, must be addressed at political level (FG3, AN, 361–68; Gilmore & Khosla, 2020). Policymakers are responsible for implementing a FGHP and creating an enabling environment. Policy processes must be accompanied by civil society (FG1, SE + A, 709–19; Gupta et al., 2019).

However, altering established structures requires profound considerations to ensure for sustainable alternatives. As with any endeavour related to feminism or global health, dominant knowledge paradigms must be questioned and reconsidered (FG2, SM, 684–95). This implies a radical transformation of the status

© The Author(s), under exclusive license to Springer Fachmedien Wiesbaden GmbH, part of Springer Nature 2023
H. Eger, *Feminist Global Health Policy*, BestMasters,
https://doi.org/10.1007/978-3-658-43497-7_8

quo—a demanding but necessary shift (FG2, OLU, 515–20). Devolving leadership to people who are rooted in the community allows for sensitive and meaningful change that is responsive to people's needs (FG2, SM, 712–19; Heymann et al., 2019). Participation and inclusion of various standpoints and acknowledging subjectivity, as identified important for a FGHP, also proved valuable in the conduct of this research in order to obtain meaningful findings.

This framework is intended as a global document, in alignment with the objective of this thesis. The universal scope allows for implementation in different settings. The flexibility of the framework facilitates context-specific adaption to encounter particular health-related challenges. Policymakers and researchers are encouraged to adopt and test the framework. Future research should be conducted in diverse settings to examine, on the one hand, the consistency of the universal principles and, on the other hand, the flexibility of the framework and potential modifications. Orientation to an intersectional, decolonial approach should direct research as well as policy processes. This implies that there does not exist one universal solution. Those in power must reflect on knowledge paradigms and power dynamics. Discouragement among policymakers can be avoided by embarking on this process together with the community and continuous awareness raising at all levels. Listening to marginalised people enables a shift in mindsets and power towards better health for all.

Current developments reveal that we are far from reaching that objective. Nevertheless, it is essential to not lose hope, to turn the vision into lived experience one day. Because collectively, change is possible.

*And if we want to achieve our goal, then let us empower ourselves with the weapon of knowledge and let us shield ourselves with unity and togetherness.*

(Malala Yousafzai, 2013)

# References

Abimbola, S., & Pai, M. (2020). Will global health survive its decolonisation? *The Lancet, 396*(10263), 1627–1628.

Aboelela, S. W., Larson, E., Bakken, S., Carrasquillo, O., Formicola, A., Glied, S. A., Haas, J., & Gebbie, K. M. (2007). Defining interdisciplinary research: Conclusions from a critical review of the literature. *Health Services Research, 42*(1, Part 1), 329–346.

Adepoju, P. (2022). Sexual Exploitation and Abuse Cloud Still Hovers over WHO as WHA75 Kicks Off. *Health Policy Watch, 23.05.2022*. Retrieved from: https://healthpolicy-watch. news/sexual-exploitation-abuse-who-wha75/ [28.06.2022]

Affun-Adegbulu, C., & Adegbulu, O. (2020). Decolonising Global (Public) Health: From Western universalism to Global pluriversalities. *BMJ Global Health, 5,* e002947.

African Union (AU) (2019). *AU Strategy for Gender Equality & Women's Empowerment 2018–2028.* Addis Ababa: AU.

Alencar Albuquerque, G., Lima Garcia, C. de, Da Silva Quirino, G., Alves, M. J. H., Belém, J. M., dos Santos Figueiredo, Francisco Winter, Da Silva Paiva, L., do Nascimento, V. B., Da Silva Maciel, É., Valenti, V. E., Abreu, L. C. de, & Adami, F. (2016). Access to health services by lesbian, gay, bisexual, and transgender persons: Systematic literature review. *BMC International Health and Human Rights, 16*(1), 2.

Allotey, P., Remme, M., & Lo, S. (2019). Doing gender better: can the UN step up? *The Lancet, 393*(10189), 2371–2373.

Arruzza, C., Bhattacharya, T., & Fraser, N. (2019). *Feminism for the 99 percent: A manifesto.* London, New York: Verso.

Barone, C. (1999). Bringing Classism Into The Race & Gender Picture. *Race, Gender & Class, 6*(3), 5–32.

Barre, A., Gordon, A., de la Plaza, C., Cortés Valderrama, G., Niazi, M., & Spitzer, P. (2022). Gender just climate solutions. WECF & WGC. Retrieved from: https://womeng enderclimate.org/wp-content/uploads/2022/11/WGC-brochure-EN_2022-11-03_web. pdf [16.11.2022]

Becker, M. (1999). Patriarchy and Inequality: Towards a Substantive Feminism. *University of Chicago Legal Forum, 1*(3), 21–88.

Beijing Declaration and Platform for Action (1995). Fourth World Conference on Women, 15 September 1995, A/CONF.177/20 (1995) and A/CONF.177/20/Add.1 (1995).

Benjeaa,Y., & Geysels, Y. (2020). Gender bias in the clinical evaluation of effectiveness in therapies. *Applied Clinical Trials, 29*(12), 30–33.

Bernarding, N., Lunz, K., Anderson, S., & Baskakov, A. (2021). *Make Foreign Policy Feminist. A Feminist Foreign Policy Manifesto for Germany.* Berlin: CFFP.

Blatter, J., Langer, P. C., & Wagemann, C. (2018). *Qualitative Methoden in der Politikwissenschaft: Eine Einführung.* Wiesbaden: Springer.

Bracke, P., Delaruelle, K., Dereuddre, R., & van de Velde, S. (2020). Depression in women and men, cumulative disadvantage and gender inequality in 29 European countries. *Social Science & Medicine, 267,* 113354.

Brinkmann, U., Dörre, K., Röbenack, S., Kraemer, K., & Speidel, F. (2006). *Prekäre Arbeit: Ursachen, Ausmaß, soziale Folgen und subjektive Verarbeitungsformen unsicherer Beschäftigungsverhältnisse. Gesprächskreis Migration und Integration.* Bonn: Friedrich-Ebert-Stiftung.

Bryman, A. (2016). *Social research methods* (Fifth edition). Oxford: Oxford University Press.

Butler, J. (1999). *Gender Trouble: Feminism and the subversion of identity.* New York: Routledge.

Büyüm, A. M., Kenney, C., Koris, A., Mkumba, L., & Raveendran, Y. (2020). Decolonising global health: If not now, when? *BMJ Global Health, 5,* e003394.

Canto, J. G., Rogers, W. J., Goldberg, R. J., Peterson, E. D., Wenger, N. K., Vaccarino, V., Kiefe, C. I., Frederick, P. D., Sopko, G., & Zheng, Z.-J. (2012). Association of Age and Sex With Myocardial Infarction Symptom Presentation and In-Hospital Mortality. *JAMA, 307*(8), 813–822.

Carastathis, A. (2014). The Concept of Intersectionality in Feminist Theory. *Philosophy Compass, 9*(5), 304–314.

Centola, D., Guilbeault, D., Sarkar, U., Khoong, E., & Zhang, J. (2021). The reduction of race and gender bias in clinical treatment recommendations using clinician peer networks in an experimental setting. *Nature Communications, 12,* 6585.

CFFP. (2021). *A Feminist Global Health Policy: A Centre for Feminist Foreign Policy Briefing.* Berlin: CFFP.

Chancel, L., Piketty, T., Saez, E., & Zucman, G. (2021). *World Inequality Report 2022.* Paris: World Inequality Lab.

Cislaghi, B., & Heise, L. (2020). Gender norms and social norms: Differences, similarities and why they matter in prevention science. *Sociology of Health & Illness, 42*(2), 407–422.

Connell, R. W. (1990). The State, Gender, and Sexual Politics: Theory and Appraisal. *Theory and Society, 19*(5), 507–544.

Convention on the Elimination of All Forms of Discrimination against Women. Adopted and opened for signature, ratification and accession by General Assembly resolution 34/180 of 18 December 1979 entry into force 3 September 1981, in accordance with article 27(1), 1979.

Cook, J. A., & Fonow, M. M. (2019). Knowledge and women's interests: Issues of epistemology and methodology in feminist sociological research. In J. M. Nielsen (Ed.), *Feminist Research Methods: Exemplary Readings in the Social Sciences* (pp. 69–93). London: Routledge.

Council of Europe Convention on preventing and combating violence against women and domestic violence Istanbul, 11.V.2011.

Courtenay, W. H. (2000). Constructions of masculinity and their influence on men's well-being: a theory of gender and health. *Social Science & Medicine, 50*(10), 1385–1401.

Crenshaw, K. (1989). Demarginalizing the Intersection of Race and Sex: A Black Feminist Critique of Antidiscrimination Doctrine, Feminist Theory and Antiracist Politics. *University of Chicago Legal Forum, 1*(8), 139–167.

CSDH. (2008). *Closing the gap in a generation: health equity through action on the social determinants of health. Final Report of the Commission on Social Determinants of Health.* Geneva: WHO.

Cyba, E. (2010). Patriarchat: Wandel und Aktualität. In R. Becker & B. Kortendiek (Eds.), *Handbuch Frauen- und Geschlechterforschung: Theorie, Methoden, Empirie* (pp. 17–22). Wiesbaden: Springer VS.

Davies, S. E., Harman, S., Manjoo, R., Tanyag, M., & Wenham, C. (2019). Why it must be a feminist global health agenda. *The Lancet, 393*(10171), 601–603.

Davis, A. Y. (1981). *Women, race and class.* London: Penguin Books.

Davis, A. Y. (2016). *Freedom Is a Constant Struggle. Ferguson, Palestine, and the Foundations of a Movement.* Chicago: Haymarket Books.

de Lima Costa, C. (2016). Gender and Equivocation: Notes on Decolonial Feminist Translations. In W. Harcourt (Ed.), *The Palgrave Handbook of Gender and Development* (pp. 48–61). London: Palgrave Macmillan.

Deacon, B. (2007). *Global social policy & governance.* London: SAGE.

Declaration of Alma-Ata (1978). International Conference on Primary Health Care, Alma-Ata, USSR, 6–12 September 1978.

Deivanayagam, T. A., Selvarajah, S., Hickel, J., Guinto, R. R., Morais Sato, P. de, Bonifacio, J., English, S., Huq, M., Issa, R., Mulindwa, H., Nagginda, H. P., Sharma, C., & Devakumar, D. (2022). Climate change, health, and discrimination: action towards racial justice. *The Lancet, online first* (4 Nov 2022).

Deutsche Gesetzliche Unfallversicherung (DGUV) (2021). *Arbeitsunfallgeschehen 2020.* Berlin: DGUV.

Deutsche Gesellschaft für die Vereinten Nationen e.V. (DGVN) (n.d.): Das System der Vereinten Nationen. Retrieved from: https://dgvn.de/fileadmin/user_upload/DOKUMENTE/DGVN_UN_Systemuebersicht.pdf [30.07.2022]

Dhatt, R., & Pley, C. (2021). Gender and Global Health Inequality. In R. Haring, I. Kickbusch, D. Ganten, & M. Moeti (Eds.), *Handbook of Global Health* (pp. 1145–1191). Cham: Springer.

Dill, B. T., & Kohlman, M. H. (2012). Intersectionality: A Transformative Paradigm in Feminist Theory and Social Justice. In S. Hesse-Biber (Ed.), *Handbook of Feminist Research: Theory and Praxis* (pp. 154–174). Thousand Oaks: SAGE Publications, Inc.

Dresing, T., & Pehl, T. (2018). *Praxisbuch Interview, Transkription & Analyse. Anleitungen und Regelsysteme für qualitativ Forschende.* (8. ed.). Marburg: Dr. Dresing und Pehl GmbH.

Dhawan, P., Goel, S., & Ghosh, A. (2021). Quality of life of tobacco users—A correlation with duration of use and nicotine dependence. *The Indian journal of tuberculosis, 68S,* S60–S64.

Eggers, M. M., Kilomba, G., Piesche, P., & Arndt, S. (2005). Mythen, Masken und Subjekte. Kritische Weißseinsforschung in Deutschland. Münster: UNRAST-Verlag.

EIGE (2021). *Gender Equality Index 2021: Health.* Luxembourg: Publications Office of the European Union.

European Commission (EC) (2020a). Communication from the Commission to the European Parliament, the Council, the European Economic and Social Committee and the Committee of the Regions. A Union of Equality: Gender Equality Strategy 2020 – 2025. Brussels, 5.3.2020, COM(2020) 152 final.

European Commission (EC) (2020b). *EU Gender Action Plan III. An ambitious agenda for gender equality and women's empowerment in EU external action.* Brussels: European Union.

Ford, C. L., & Airhihenbuwa, C. O. (2010). Critical Race Theory, race equity, and public health: Toward antiracism praxis. *American Journal of Public Health, 100 Suppl*(1), S30-S35.

Fulu, E., Leung, L., & Viana, M. (2021). Feminist movements are key to public health equity. *The BMJ.* Retrieved from: https://blogs.bmj.com/bmj/2021/06/28/feminist-movements-are-key-to-public-health-equity [12.07.2022]

G7 Gender Equality Advisory Council (2021). Building back better for women and girls. Report of the G7 Gender Equality Advisory Council 2021. Retrieved from: https://www.gov.uk/government/publications/report-of-the-g7-gender-equality-advisory-council-2021 [10.07.2022]

Gannon, S., & Davies, B. (2012). Postmodern, Post-Structural, and Critical Theories. In S. Hesse-Biber (Ed.), *Handbook of Feminist Research: Theory and Praxis* (pp. 65–91). Thousand Oaks: SAGE Publications, Inc.

Gilmore, K., & Khosla, R. (2020). Sex, sexuality, and sexual and reproductive health: the role of human rights. *Open Global Rights.* Retrieved from: https://www.openglobalrights.org/the-role-of-human-rights-in-sexuality-and-sexual-and-reproductive-health/ [04.07.2022]

Glick, P., & Fiske, S.T. (1997). Hostile and benevolent sexism. Measuring Ambivalent Sexist Attitudes toward women. *Psychology of Women Quarterly, 21,* 119–135.

Global Health 50/50 (2022). Boards for all? A review of power, policy and people on the boards of organisations active in global health. Retrieved from: https://globalhealth5050.org/2022-report/ [22.04.2022]

Goulimari, P. (2020). Feminist Theory. In P. Goulimari (Ed.), *Oxford Research Encyclopedia of Literature* (pp. 1–33). Oxford: Oxford University Press.

Greenwood, M., & Lindsay, N.M. (2019). A commentary on land, health, and Indigenous knowledge(s). *Global Health Promotion, 26*(3 suppl), 82–86.

Gunda-Werner-Institut, CARE Deutschland, Greenpeace, medica mondiale, IFFF Deutschland, Owen, Deutscher Frauenrat, Plan International, Polis 180, Women for Women International Deutschland, AMICA, The Canaan Project, Frauennetzwerk für Frieden, Deutscher Frauenring, UN Women Deutschland, International Rescue Committee, Deutsche Gesellschaft für die Vereinten Nationen, & CFFP. (2022). Annäherung an eine feministische Außenpolitik Deutschlands. Retrieved from: https://www.boell.de/de/2022/07/28/annaeherung-eine-feministische-aussenpolitik-deutschlands [07.11.2022]

Gupta, G. R., Oomman, N., Grown, C., Conn, K., Hawkes, S., Shawar, Y. R., Shiffman, J., Buse, K., Mehra, R., Bah, C. A., Heise, L., Greene, M. E [Margaret E.], Weber, A. M., Heymann, J., Hay, K., Raj, A., Henry, S., Klugman, J., & Darmstadt, G. L. (2019). Gender equality and gender norms: framing the opportunities for health. *The Lancet, 393*(10190), 2550–2562.

Habtezion, S. (2016). *Gender and climate change. Overview of linkages between gender and climate change.* New York: UNDP.

Haig, B. D. (1999). Feminist Research Methodology. In J. P. Keeves & G. Lakomski (Eds.), *Issues in Educational Research* (pp. 222–231). Kidlington, Oxford, New York: Pergamon/ Elsevier.

Hanefeld, J., & Fischer, H.-T. (2021). Global Health: Definition, Principles, and Drivers. In R. Haring, I. Kickbusch, D. Ganten, & M. Moeti (Eds.), *Handbook of Global Health* (pp. 3–27). Cham: Springer.

Harding, S. G. (1987). *Feminism and methodology: Social science issues.* Bloomington: Indiana Univ. Press.

Hawkes, S., & Buse, K. (2013). Gender and global health: evidence, policy, and inconvenient truths. *The Lancet, 381*(9879), 1783–1787.

Hay, K., McDougal, L., Percival, V., Henry, S., Klugman, J., Wurie, H., Raven, J., Shabalala, F., Fielding-Miller, R., Dey, A., Dehingia, N., Morgan, R., Atmavilas, Y., Saggurti, N., Yore, J., Blokhina, E., Huque, R., Barasa, E., Bhan, N., . . . Rao Gupta, G. (2019). Disrupting gender norms in health systems: making the case for change. *The Lancet, 393*(10190), 2535–2549.

Heidari, S., & Doyle, H. (2020). An Invitation to a Feminist Approach to Global Health Data. *Health and Human Rights Journal, 22*(2), 75–78.

Heinrich-Böll-Stiftung, & Fair Share (2022). Feminist Development Policy. A pathway towards feminist global collaboration. Retrieved from: https://www.boell.de/sites/default/files/2022-09/feminist_development_policy.pdf [16.11.2022]

Heise, L., Greene, M. E, Opper, N., Stavropoulou, M., Harper, C., Nascimento, M., Zewdie, D., Darmstadt, G. L., Greene, M. E., Hawkes, S., Henry, S., Heymann, J., Klugman, J., Levine, R., Raj, A., & Rao Gupta, G. (2019). Gender inequality and restrictive gender norms: framing the challenges to health. *The Lancet, 393*(10189), 2440–2454.

Herten-Crabb, A., & Davies, S. E. (2020). Why WHO needs a feminist economic agenda. *The Lancet, 395*(10229), 1018–1020.

Heymann, J., Levy, J. K., Bose, B., Ríos-Salas, V., Mekonen, Y., Swaminathan, H., Omidakhsh, N., Gadoth, A., Huh, K., Greene, M. E [Margaret E.], Darmstadt, G. L., Greene, M. E, Hawkes, S., Heise, L., Henry, S., Klugman, J., Levine, R., Raj, A., & Rao Gupta, G. (2019). Improving health with programmatic, legal, and policy approaches to reduce gender inequality and change restrictive gender norms. *The Lancet, 393*(10190), 2522–2534.

Hickel, J. (2020). Quantifying national responsibility for climate breakdown: an equality-based attribution approach for carbon dioxide emissions in excess of the planetary boundary. *The Lancet Planetary Health, 4*(9), e399–e404.

Hill Collins, P. (2000). *Black feminist thought: Knowledge, consciousness, and the politics of empowerment* (Second edition). London, New York: Routledge.

Hill Collins, P. (2019). *Intersectionality as Critical Social Theory.* Durham: Duke University Press.

hooks, b. (1982). *Ain't I a woman: Black women and feminism.* London: Pluto Press.

hooks, b. (2001). *All about love: New visions.* New York: Harper Perennial.

Hu, X., Wang, T., Huang, D., Wang, Y., & Li, Q. (2021). Impact of social class on health: The mediating role of health self-management. *PLoS ONE 16*(7), e0254692.

Irwin, R. E. (2019). Lessons from Sweden's feminist foreign policy for global health. *The Lancet, 393*(10171), e27–e28.

Jhpiego (2016). *Gender analysis toolkit for health systems.* Baltimore: Jhpiego.

John, N. A., Stoebenau, K., Ritter, S., Edmeades, J. & Balvin, N. (2017). Gender Socialization during Adolescence in Low- and Middle-Income Countries: Conceptualization, influences and outcomes. *Innocenti Discussion Paper* 2017–01, Florence: UNICEF Office of Research – Innocenti.

Kahan, J. P. (2001). Focus Groups as a Tool for Policy Analysis. *Analyses of Social Issues and Public Policy*, *1*, 129–146.

Kantola, J., & Lombardo, E. (2017). Feminist political analysis: Exploring strengths, hegemonies and limitations. *Feminist Theory*, *18*(3), 323–341.

Kapilashrami, A., & Hankivsky, O. (2018). Intersectionality and why it matters to global health. *The Lancet*, *391*(10140), 2589–2591.

Kaur, R., & Nagaich, S. (2019). Understanding Feminist Research Methodology in Social Sciences. *SSRN*, Available at: https://ssrn.com/abstract=3392500 [14.02.2022]

Khan, T., Abimbola, S., Kyobutungi, C., & Pai, M. (2022). How we classify countries and people-and why it matters. *BMJ Global Health*, *7*, e009704.

Khosla, R., Allotey, P., & Gruskin, S. (2022). Reimagining human rights in global health: what will it take? *BMJ Global Health*, *7*(8), e010373.

King, M. L. Jr. (1966). Presentation at the Second National Convention of the Medical Committee for Human Rights, Chicago, 25 March 1966.

King, T. L., Shields, M., Sojo, V., Daraganova, G., Currier, D., O'Neil, A., King, K., & Milner, A. (2020). Expressions of masculinity and associations with suicidal ideation among young males. *BMC Psychiatry*, *20*(1).

Kitzinger, J. (1995). Qualitative research. Introducing focus groups. *BMJ*, *311*, 299–302.

Kivits, J., Ricci, L., & Minary, L. (2019). Interdisciplinary research in public health: The 'why' and the 'how'. *Journal of Epidemiology and Community Health*, *73*(12), 1061–1062

Kluge, U., Aichberger, M. C., Heinz, E., Udeogu-Gözalan, C., & Abdel-Fatah, D. (2020). Rassismus und psychische Gesundheit. *Der Nervenarzt*, *91*(11), 1017–1024.

Klugman, J., Li, L., Barker, K. M., Parsons, J., & Dale, K. (2019). How are the domains of women's inclusion, justice, and security associated with maternal and infant mortality across countries? Insights from the Women, Peace, and Security Index. *SSM—Population Health*, *9*(100486).

Knight, M., Bunch, K., Tuffnell, D., Patel, R., Shakespeare, J., Kotnis, R., Kenyon, S., & Kurinczuk, J. J. (2021). *Saving Lives, Improving Mothers' Care Core report: lessons learned to inform maternity care from the UK and Ireland Confidential Enquiries into Maternal Deaths and Morbidity 2017–19*. Oxford: MBRACE-UK.

Koplan, J. P., Bond, T. C., Merson, M. H., Reddy, K. S., Rodriguez, M. H., Sewankambo, N. K., & Wasserheit, J. N. (2009). Towards a common definition of global health. *The Lancet*, *373*(9679), 1993–1995.

Kuckartz, U. (2016). *Qualitative Inhaltsanalyse. Methoden, Praxis, Computerunterstützung* (3. ed.). Weinheim: Beltz.

Kuckartz, U. (2019). Qualitative Text Analysis: A Systematic Approach. In G. Kaiser & N. Presmeg (Eds.), *ICME-13 Monographs. Compendium for Early Career Researchers in Mathematics Education* (pp. 181–197). Cham: Springer International Publishing.

Lamnek, S., & Krell, C. (2016). *Qualitative Sozialforschung* (6. ed.). Weinheim: Beltz.

Lampert, T., Hoebel, J., & Kroll, L. E. (2019). Soziale Unterschiede in der Mortalität und Lebenserwartung in Deutschland. Aktuelle Situation und Trends. *Journal of Health Monitoring*, *4*(1), 3–15.

Lampert, T., Hoebel, J., Kuntz, B., Finger, J. D., Hölling, H., Lange, M., Mauz, E., Mensink, G., Poethko-Müller, C., Schienkiewitz, A., Starker, A., Zeiher, J., & Kurth, B.-M. (2019). Gesundheitliche Ungleichheiten bei Kindern und Jugendlichen in Deutschland – Zeitliche Entwicklung und Trends der KiGGS-Studie. *Journal of Health Monitoring, 4*(1), 16–40.

Lampert, T., Kroll, L. E., Kuntz, B., & Hoebel, J. (2018). Gesundheitliche Ungleichheit in Deutschland und im internationalen Vergleich: Zeitliche Entwicklungen und Trends. *Journal of Health Monitoring, 3*(S1), 2–25.

Lessenich, S. (2018). *Neben uns die Sintflut: Wie wir auf Kosten anderer leben.* München: Piper.

Liamputtong, P., & Rice, Z. S. (2021). Qualitative Research in Global Health Research. In R. Haring, I. Kickbusch, D. Ganten, & M. Moeti (Eds.), *Handbook of Global Health* (pp. 213–238). Cham: Springer.

Liu ,K.A., & DiPietro Mager, N.A. (2016). Women's involvement in clinical trials: historical perspective and future implications. *Pharmacy Practice, 14*(1), 708.

Lorde, A. (1984). *Sister Outsider.* New York: Crossing Press.

Lugones, M. (2016). The Coloniality of Gender. In W. Harcourt (Ed.), *The Palgrave Handbook of Gender and Development* (pp. 13–33). London: Palgrave Macmillan.

Lundberg, O., Dahl, E., Fritzell, J., Palme, J., & Sjöberg, O. (2016). *Social protection, income and health inequities. Final report of the Task Group on GDP, Taxes, Income and Welfare: Review of social determinants of health and the health divide in the WHO European Region.* Copenhagen: WHO Regional Office for Europe.

Lunz, K. (2022). *Die Zukunft der Aussenpolitik ist feministisch: Wie globale Krisen gelöst werden müssen.* Berlin: Econ.

Mackenbach, J.P. (2006). *Health Inequalities: Europe in Profile.* Rotterdam: Erasmus MC.

Mair, S., Jones, A., Ward, J., Christie, I., Druckman, A., & Lyon, F. (2017). A critical review of the role of indicators in implementing the sustainable development goals. In W. L. Filho (Ed.), *Handbook of sustainability science and research* (pp. 41– 56 ). Cham: Springer.

March of Dimes (2019). *2019 March of Dimes Report Card. Health Moms. Strong Babies.* Arlington: March of Dimes.

Markham, S., & Foster, S. (2021). Gender equality is fundamental to promoting democracy. *Just Security.* Retrieved from: https://www.justsecurity.org/75681/gender-equality-is-fundamental-to-promoting-democracy/ [05.02.2022]

Marmot, M., & Allen, J. J. (2014). Social determinants of health equity. *American Journal of Public Health, 104*(Suppl 4), S517–S519.

Maruska, J. H. (2017). *Feminist Ontologies, Epistemologies, Methodologies, and Methods in International Relations. Oxford Research Encyclopedia of International Studies.* (Vol. 1). Oxford: Oxford University Press.

McCoy, D., & Hilson, M. (2009). Civil society, its organizations, and global health governance. In K. Buse, W. Hein, & N. Drager (Eds.), *Making sense of global health governance: A policy perspective* (pp. 209–231). Basingstoke: Palgrave Macmillan.

McHugh, M. C. (2014). Feminist Qualitative Research: Toward Transformation of Science and Society. In P. Leavy & M. C. McHugh (Eds.), *The Oxford Handbook of Qualitative Research* (pp. 136–164). Oxford: Oxford University Press.

McMaughan, D. J., Oloruntoba, O., & Smith, M. L. (2020). Socioeconomic Status and Access to Healthcare: Interrelated Drivers for Healthy Aging. *Frontiers in Public Health*, *8*(231).

Medina-Martínez, J., Saus-Ortega, C., Sánchez-Lorente, M. M., Sosa-Palanca, E. M., García-Martínez, P., & Mármol-López, M. I. (2021). Health Inequities in LGBT People and Nursing Interventions to Reduce Them: A Systematic Review. *International Journal of Environmental Research and Public Health*, *18*(22).

Mesman, J., & Groeneveld, M. G. (2018). Gendered parenting in early childhood: Subtle but unmistakable if you know where to look. *Child development perspectives*, *12*(1), 22–27.

Meyer, O. L., Castro-Schilo, L., & Aguilar-Gaxiola, S. (2014). Determinants of mental health and self-rated health: A model of socioeconomic status, neighborhood safety, and physical activity. *American Journal of Public Health*, *104*(9), 1734–1741.

Miles, R. (1991). *Rassismus: Einführung in die Geschichte und Theorie eines Begriffs*. Hamburg: Argument Verlag.

Miller, S., Wherry, L. R., & Foster, D. G. (2020a). What happens after an abortion denial? A Review of Results from the Turnaway Study. January 2020. *AEA Papers and Proceedings*, *110*, 226–230.

Miller, S., Wherry, L.R., Foster, D.G. (2020b) The economic consequences of being denied an abortion. January 2020. *NBER Working Paper Series*, Working Paper 26662, National Bureau of Economic Research.

Mohamed, S. (2022). Diversity Ars Culture. Schwarz. Available at: https://diversity-arts-cul ture.berlin/woerterbuch/schwarz [23.11.2022]

Mukhopadhyay, M. (2016). Mainstreaming Gender or "Streaming" Gender Away: Feminists Marooned in the Development Business. In W. Harcourt (Ed.), *The Palgrave Handbook of Gender and Development* (pp. 77–91). London: Palgrave Macmillan.

Nash, C. J. (2020). Patriarchy. In A. Kobayashi (Ed.), *International Encyclopedia of Human Geography* (pp. 43–47). San Diego: Elsevier.

Nettleton, C., Stephens, C., Bristow, F., Claro S., Hart, T., McCausland, C., & Mijlof, I. (2007). Utz Wachil: Findings from an International Study of Indigenous Perspectives on Health and Environment. *EcoHealth*, *4*, 461–471.

Newman, C., Chama, P. K., Mugisha, M., Matsiko, C. W., & Oketcho, V. (2017). Reasons behind current gender imbalances in senior global health roles and the practice and policy changes that can catalyze organizational change. *Global Health, Epidemiology and Genomics*, *2*(e19), 1–26.

Noonan, A. S., Velasco-Mondragon, H. E., & Wagner, F. A. (2016). Improving the health of African Americans in the USA: An overdue opportunity for social justice. *Public Health Reviews*, *37*(1), 12.

Olmos-Vega, F. M., Stalmeijer, R. E., Varpio, L., & Kahlke, R. (2022). A practical guide to reflexivity in qualitative research: Amee Guide No. 149. *Medical Teacher*, 1–11.

Padberg, B. (2014). The Center for Interdisciplinary Research (ZiF)— Epistemic and Institutional Considerations. In B. Padberg & P. Weingart (Eds.), *University experiments in interdisciplinarity: Obstacles and opportunities* (pp. 95–114). Bielefeld: Transcript.

Palència, L., Moortel, D. de, Artazcoz, L., Salvador-Piedrafita, M., Puig-Barrachina, V., Hagqvist, E., Pérez, G., Ruiz, M. E., Trujillo-Alemán, S., Vanroelen, C., Malmusi, D., & Borrell, C. (2017). Gender Policies and Gender Inequalities in Health in Europe: Results of the SOPHIE Project. *International Journal of Health Services*, *47*(1), 61–82.

Paradies, Y., Ben, J., Denson, N., Elias, A., Priest, N., Pieterse, A., Gupta, A., Kelaher, M., & Gee, G. (2015). Racism as a Determinant of Health: A Systematic Review and Meta-Analysis. *PLOS ONE, 10*(9), e0138511.

Parker, R., & Aggleton, P. (2003). HIV and AIDS-related stigma and discrimination: a conceptual framework and implications for action. *Social Science & Medicine, 57*(1), 13–24.

Permanyer, I., & Spijker, J. (2021). Socioeconomics and the Macro- and Micro-Level Determinants of Global Health Inequality. In R. Haring, I. Kickbusch, D. Ganten, & M. Moeti (Eds.), *Handbook of Global Health* (pp. 1091–1126). Cham: Springer.

People's Health Movement, Medact, Third World Network, Health Poverty Action, Medico International, ALAMES, Viva Salud, & SAMA (2022). *Global Health Watch 6. In the shadow of the pandemic.* London: Bloomsbury Academic.

Petchesky, R. P. (2016). Gendered Well-Being. Globalization, Women's Health and Economic Justice: Reflections Post-September 11. In W. Harcourt (Ed.), *The Palgrave Handbook of Gender and Development* (pp. 145–172). London: Palgrave Macmillan.

Phillips, S. P. (2005). Defining and measuring gender: A social determinant of health whose time has come. *International Journal for Equity in Health, 4*(11).

Ray, D., & Linden, M. (2018). Health, inequality and income: a global study using simultaneous model. *Economic Structures, 7*(22).

Reisner, S. L., Poteat, T., Keatley, J., Cabral, M., Mothopeng, T., Dunham, E., Holland, C. E., Max, R., & Baral, S. D. (2016). Global health burden and needs of transgender populations: a review. *The Lancet, 388*(10042), 412–436.

Rogers, W. A. (2006). Feminism and public health ethics. *Journal of Medical Ethics, 32*(6), 351–354.

Roig, E. (2021). *Why We Matter: Das Ende der Unterdrückung.* Berlin: Aufbau digital.

Rommel, A., Saß, A. C., Born, S., & Ellert, U. (2015). Die gesundheitliche Lage von Menschen mit Migrationshintergrund und die Bedeutung des sozioökonomischen Status : Erste Ergebnisse der Studie zur Gesundheit Erwachsener in Deutschland (DEGS1). *Bundesgesundheitsblatt, Gesundheitsforschung, Gesundheitsschutz, 58*(6), 543–552.

Ross, L., & Solinger, R. (2017). *Reproductive Justice: An Introduction.* Berkeley: University of California Press.

Safaei, J. (2012). Democracy, Human Rights and Women's Health. *Mens Sana Monographs, 10*(1), 134–142.

Sardinha, L., Maheu-Giroux, M., Stöckl, H., Meyer, S. R., & García-Moreno, C. (2022). Global, regional, and national prevalence estimates of physical or sexual, or both, intimate partner violence against women in 2018. *The Lancet, 399*(10327), 803–813.

Scambler, G. (2019). Sociology, Social Class, Health Inequalities, and the Avoidance of "Classism". *Frontiers in Sociology, 4*(56).

Scherr, A. (2016). *Diskriminierung* (2. ed.). Wiesbaden: Springer VS.

Schwingshackl, L., Lampousi, A. M., Portillo, M. P., Romaguera, D., Hoffmann, G., & Boeing, H. (2017). Olive oil in the prevention and management of type 2 diabetes mellitus: a systematic review and meta-analysis of cohort studies and intervention trials. *Nutrition & diabetes, 7*(4), e262.

Sen, G., Govender, V., & El-Gamal, S. (2020). *Universal health coverage, gender equality and social protection: A health systems approach.* New York: UN Women.

Sen, G., Iyer, A., Chattopadhyay, S., & Khosla, R. (2020). When accountability meets power: Realizing sexual and reproductive health and rights. *International Journal for Equity in Health, 19*(111).

Shawky, S. (2021). Geography of Economic Disparities and Global Health Inequality. In R. Haring, I. Kickbusch, D. Ganten, & M. Moeti (Eds.), *Handbook of Global Health* (pp. 1215–1228). Cham: Springer.

Solar, O., & Irwin, A. (2010). *A conceptual framework for action on the social determinants of health. Social Determinants of Health Discussion Paper 2 (Policy and Practice)*. Geneva: WHO.

Springer, K. W., Hankivsky, O., & Bates, L. M. (2012). Gender and health: Relational, intersectional, and biosocial approaches. *Social Science & Medicine, 74*(11), 1661–1666.

Sridharan, S., Maplazi, J., Shirodkar, A., Richardson, E., & Nakaima, A. (2016). Incorporating gender, equity, and human rights into the action planning process: Moving from rhetoric to action. *Global Health Action, 9*(30870), 1–12.

Stanley, L. (2016). Using focus groups in political science and international relations. *Politics, 36*(3), 236–249.

Starrs, A. M., Ezeh, A. C., Barker, G., Basu, A., Bertrand, J. T., Blum, R., Coll-Seck, A. M., Grover, A., Laski, L., Roa, M., Sathar, Z. A., Say, L., Serour, G. I., Singh, S., Stenberg, K., Temmerman, M., Biddlecom, A., Popinchalk, A., Summers, C., & Ashford, L. S. (2018). Accelerate progress—sexual and reproductive health and rights for all: report of the Guttmacher– Lancet Commission. *The Lancet, 391*(10140), 2642–2692.

Stiftung Gesundheitswissen (2020). *Statussymbol Gesundheit. Wie sich der soziale Status auf Prävention und Gesundheit auswirken kann*. Berlin: Stiftung Gesundheitswissen.

Tausch, A. P., & Menold, N. (2015). *Methodische Aspekte der Durchführung von Fokusgruppen in der Gesundheitsforschung: Welche Anforderungen ergeben sich aufgrund der besonderen Zielgruppen und Fragestellungen?* (GESIS Papers). Köln: GESIS—Leibniz-Institut für Sozialwissenschaften.

Teixeira da Silva, J. A. (2021). Rethinking the use of the term 'Global South' in academic publishing. *European Science Editing, 47*, e67829.

Tolhurst, R., Leach, B., Price, J., Robinson, J., Ettore, E., Scott-Samuel, A., Kilonzo, N., Sabuni, L. P., Robertson, S., Kapilashrami, A., Bristow, K., Lang, R., Romao, F., & Theobald, S. (2012). Intersectionality and gender mainstreaming in international health: Using a feminist participatory action research process to analyse voices and debates from the global south and north. *Social Science & Medicine, 74*(11), 1825–1832.

Tracy, S. J. (2010). Qualitative Quality: Eight "Big-Tent" Criteria for Excellent Qualitative Research. *Qualitative Inquiry, 16*(10), 837–851.

United Nations (UN) (1965). International Convention on the Elimination of All Forms of Racial Discrimination. Adopted and opened for signature and ratification by General Assembly resolution 2106 (XX) of 21 December 1965, entry into force 4 January 1969, in accordance with Article 19.

United Nation (UN) (2015a). Action against gender-related killing of women and girls. Report of the Secretary-General. A/70/93

United Nations (UN) (2015b). Transforming our world: the 2030 Agenda for Sustainable Development: Resolution adopted by the General Assembly on 25 September 2015, Seventieth session Agenda items 15 and 116, A/RES/70/1.

United Nations (UN) (2021). The United Nations System. Retrieved from: https://www.un. org/en/pdfs/un_system_chart.pdf [30.07.2022]

UNDP (2022a). The SDGs in Action. Retrieved from: https://www.undp.org/sustainable-dev elopment-goals [30.07.2022]

UNDP (2022b). *UNDP Gender Equality Strategy 2022–2025*. New York: UNDP

UNFPA (2005). Frequently asked questions about gender equality. Retrieved from: https://www.unfpa.org/resources/frequently-asked-questions-about-gender-equality [12.04.2022]

UNFPA (2022). About us. Retrieved from: https://www.unfpa.org/about-us [30.07.2022]

United Nations Office on Drugs and Crime (UNODC) (2021). *Killings of women and girls by their intimate partner or other family members Global estimates 2020*. Vienna: UNODC

UN Women (2020). *Political declaration. On the occasion of the twenty-fifth anniversary of the fourth world conference on women*. New York: UN Women

UN Women (2022a). About us. Retrieved from: https://www.unwomen.org/en/about-us/ about-un-women [30.07.2022]

UN Women (2022b). World Conferences on Women. Retrieved from: https://www.unw omen.org/en/how-we-work/intergovernmental-support/world-conferences-on-women [12.07.2022]

Urban, H.-J. (2009). Die Mosaik-Linke. *Blätter für deutsche und internationale Politik, 5*, 71–78.

van Daalen, K.R., Kaiser, J., Kebede, S., Cipriano, G., Maimouni, H., Olumese, E., Chui, A., Kuhn, I., & Oliver-Williams, C. (2022). Racial discrimination and adverse pregnancy outcomes: a systematic review and meta-analysis. *BMJ Global Health, 7*, e009227.

Varkey, P., Mbbs, Kureshi, S., & Lesnick, T. (2010). Empowerment of women and its association with the health of the community. *Journal of Women's Health, 19*(1), 71–76.

VENRO. (2022). *Erwartungen an eine feministische Entwicklungspolitik*. Berlin: VENRO. *Retrieved from:* https://venro.org/fileadmin/user_upload/Dateien/Daten/Publikationen/ Stellungnahmen/VENRO_Stellungnahme_Feministische_Entwicklungspolitik_2022. pdf *[07.11.2022]*

Wallerstein, I. (1974). *The Modern World System I*. New York: Academic Publishers.

Weber, A. M., Cislaghi, B., Meausoone, V., Abdalla, S., Mejía-Guevara, I., Loftus, P., Hallgren, E., Seff, I., Stark, L., Victora, C. G., Buffarini, R., Barros, A. J. D., Domingue, B. W., Bhushan, D., Gupta, R., Nagata, J. M., Shakya, H. B., Richter, L. M., Norris, S. A., . . . Rao Gupta, G. (2019). Gender norms and health: insights from global survey data. *The Lancet, 393*(10189), 2455–2468.

Wenham, C., & Davies, S. E. (2021). WHO runs the world – (not) girls: gender neglect during global health emergencies. *International Feminist Journal of Politics, 24*(3), 415–438.

Westkott, M. (2019). Feminist criticism of the social sciences. In J. M. Nielsen (Ed.), *Feminist Research Methods: Exemplary Readings in the Social Sciences* (pp. 58–68). London: Routledge.

Whitehead, M., & Burström, B. (2021). History lessons for tackling inequalities in health. *SSM Popul Health, 25*(16), 100980.

World Health Organization (WHO) (1946). Constitution of the World Health Organization. New York, 22 July 1946.

World Health Organization (WHO) (2001). WHO's contribution to the World Conference against Racism, Racial Discrimination, Xenophobia and Related Intolerance: Health and freedom from discrimination. Geneva: World Health Organization.

World Health Organization (WHO) (2014). *Gender, climate change and health.* Geneva: World Health Organization.

World Health Organization (WHO) (2016). *Innov8: Approach for reviewing national health programmes to leave no one behind: technical handbook.* Geneva: World Health Organization.

World Health Organization (WHO) (2019a). *Delivered by women, led by men: A gender and equity analysis of the global health and social workforce.* Geneva: World Health Organization.

World Health Organization (WHO) (2019b). *Primary Health Care on the Road to Universal Health Coverage: 2019 Monitoring Report.* Geneva: WHO.

World Health Organization (WHO) (2020). *Incorporating intersectional gender analysis into research on infectious diseases of poverty: a toolkit for health researchers.* Geneva: WHO.

World Health Organization (WHO) (2021). World Health Organization Headquarters. Retrieved from: https://cdn.who.int/media/docs/default-source/documents/about-us/who-hq-organigram.pdf [06.09.2022]

World Health Organization (WHO) (2022). Social determinants of health. Retrieved from: https://www.who.int/health-topics/social-determinants-of-health [15.05.2022]

Wigginton, B., & Lafrance, M. N. (2019). Learning critical feminist research: A brief introduction to feminist epistemologies and methodologies. *Feminism & Psychology, 0*(0), 1–17.

Wilkinson, R., & Marmot, M. (2004). *Soziale Determinanten von Gesundheit: Die Fakten. Gesunde Städte im 21. Jh.* (2. ed.). Kopenhagen: WHO Regional Office for Europe.

Wilkinson, R., & Pickett, K. (2010). *The spirit level. Why equality is better for everyone.* London: Penguin Books.

Wilkinson, S. (1988). The role of reflexivity in feminist psychology. *Women's Studies International Forum, 11*(5), 493–502.

Wilkinson, S. (1999). Focus Groups: A feminist method. *Psychology of Women Quarterly, 23*(2), 221–244.

Williams, A., Lyeo, J. S., Geffros, S., & Mouriopoulos, A. (2021). The integration of sex and gender considerations in health policymaking: A scoping review. *International Journal for Equity in Health, 20*(69).

Williams, D. R. (2018). Stress and the Mental Health of Populations of Color: Advancing Our Understanding of Race-related Stressors. *Journal of Health and Social Behavior, 59*(4), 466–485.

Wilson, C., & Cariola, L. A. (2020). Lgbtqi+ Youth and Mental Health: A Systematic Review of Qualitative Research. *Adolescent Research Review, 5*(2), 187–211.

Winker, G. (2015). *Care Revolution. Schritte in eine solidarische Gesellschaft.* Bielefeld: transcript.

Winter, S., Diamond, M., Green, J., Karasic, D., Reed, T., Whittle, S., & Wylie, K. (2016). Transgender people: health at the margins of society. *The Lancet, 388*(10042), 390–400.

Wright, M. T. (2021). Partizipative Gesundheitsforschung: Ursprünge und heutiger Stand. *Bundesgesundheitsblatt, Gesundheitsforschung, Gesundheitsschutz, 64*(2), 140–145,

Wu, X. Y., Han, L. H., Zhang, J. H., Luo, S., Hu, J. W., & Sun, K. (2017). The influence of physical activity, sedentary behavior on health-related quality of life among the general population of children and adolescents: A systematic review. *PloS one, 12*(11), e0187668.

Yam, E. A., Silva, M., Ranganathan, M., White, J., Hope, T. M., & Ford, C. L. (2021). Time to take critical race theory seriously: moving beyond a colour-blind gender lens in global health. *The Lancet Global Health, 9*(4), e389-e390.

Yao, Q., Li, X., Luo, F., Yang, L., & Sun, J. (2019). The historical roots and seminal research on health equity: a referenced publication year spectroscopy (RPYS) analysis. *Int J Equity Health,* 18(152).

Yousafzai, M. (2013). Malala Yousafzai: 16th birthday speech at the United Nations. Malala Fund. Retrieved from: https://malala.org/newsroom/malala-un-speech [01.12.2022]

Yuval-Davis, N. (2016). Power, Intersectionality and the Politics of Belonging. In W. Harcourt (Ed.), *The Palgrave Handbook of Gender and Development* (pp. 367–381). London: Palgrave Macmillan.

Zhou, S., Da, S., Guo, H., & Zhang, X. (2018). Work–Family Conflict and Mental Health Among Female Employees: A Sequential Mediation Model via Negative Affect and Perceived Stress. *Frontiers in Psychology, 9*(544).

# GPSR Compliance

*The European Union's (EU) General Product Safety Regulation (GPSR) is a set of rules that requires consumer products to be safe and our obligations to ensure this.*

*If you have any concerns about our products, you can contact us on ProductSafety@springernature.com*

In case Publisher is established outside the EU, the EU authorized representative is:

Springer Nature Customer Service Center GmbH
Europaplatz 3
69115 Heidelberg, Germany

The manufacturer's authorised representative in the EU is Springer
Nature Customer Service Centre GmbH, Europaplatz 3, 69115 Heidelberg,
Germany. If you have any concerns regarding our products, please
contact ProductSafety@springernature.com

Printed and bound by CPI Group (UK) Ltd, Croydon, CR0 4YY
24/04/2026
02096353-0001